I0090632

# INTERMITTENT FASTING + KETO DIET
## and Exercise Plan
## (3 IN 1 VALUE BUNDLE)

Complete Beginners Guide to Ketogenic Diet, Keto Meal Prep, Intermittent Fasting for Woman and Exercise Guide for weight loss

**SUSAN KATZ**

© **Copyright 2019 – Susan Katz All rights reserved.**

The content within this book may not be reproduced, duplicated or transmitted without direct written permission from the author or the publisher.

Under no circumstances will any blame or legal responsibility be held against the publisher, or author, for any damages, reparation, or monetary loss due to the information contained within this book. Either directly or indirectly.

Legal Notice:

This book is copyright protected. This book is only for personal use. You cannot amend, distribute, sell, use, quote or paraphrase any part, or the content within this book, without the consent of the author or publisher.

Disclaimer Notice:

Please note the information contained within this document is for educational and entertainment purposes only. All effort has been executed to present accurate, up to date, and reliable, complete information. No warranties of any kind are declared or implied. Readers acknowledge that the author is not engaging in the rendering of legal, financial, medical or professional advice. The content within this book has been derived from various sources. Please consult a licensed professional before attempting any techniques outlined in this book.

By reading this document, the reader agrees that under no circumstances are is the author responsible for any losses, direct or indirect, which are incurred as a result of the use of information contained within this document, including, but not limited to, —errors, omissions, or inaccuracies.

# 3 BOOK VALUE BUNDLE

# TABLE OF CONTENTS

## Intermittent Fasting for Women 30-Day Challenge

# Ketogenic Diet and Exercise Plan

Burn fat, gain muscle, have more energy
with simple keto meal prep

# Introduction

Burn 15 pounds in 20 minutes every day! No work needed! Try this weird trick that tricks your body into burning fat!

How many of us have seen some version of the above ad while browsing the internet? How many of us have been unfortunate enough to actually believe its claims and ended up clicking on it? Losing weight and being physically fit is one of the top wishes everybody has no matter where they're from. Like everything else, choosing the correct way to go about things is daunting just because there's so much information out there. There's a ton of evidence to support something and just as much, seemingly, which refute it. Then there is the litany of terms one needs to become familiar with when adopting any new diet plan or information.

Paleo, Keto, LCHF, HCLF, Atkins, Weight Watchers, South Beach, No carbs after 6 PM, carbs only after 6 PM, cardio vs strength training, training on an empty stomach, protein, carbs, fat.....and on and on it goes. Even if you do become comfortable with all these terms, losing weight isn't guaranteed. You might see some results but making sure the results remain is another matter entirely.

Funnily enough, it is the very existence of so many diet plans and training programs that spawn newer, shinier diets. People are always searching for a better, more "guaranteed" plan and naturally, the market rises to fill their needs. These days, given the number of content channels out there, its easy to be bombarded with media on pretty much any topic of your choice, no matter how bizarre. Even as we speak, there are probably videos being uploaded out there detailing how you can lose weight using telekinesis or some such.

Vegans and vegetarians face further issues since a lot of diets readily assume their audience has no problem consuming meat and dairy. Generally speaking, following a diet plan while living a vegan lifestyle is difficult enough and all this additional confusion is the last thing you need. How did food become so complicated? More importantly, how does one unravel it?

# BACK TO BASICS

The answer is simple: Ignore the noise and head back to the basics. Our bodies are far more resilient than we give them credit for and there is no need to treat them like porcelain dolls (assuming you don't have a debilitating disease of course). You don't need an extremely fancy diet which causes you to worry about what to and what not to eat constantly. You just need to learn some basics about how the body burns food as fuel and how by understanding this process and following some simple principles, you can make any diet work.

The Ketogenic diet is one of those basic diet plans, believe it or not. The name for this diet might be newfangled but the principles of this diet have existed in some form or another for a long time. Why? Because it's common sense! There's nothing fancy about it unless you wish to make it so.

This book is going to give you the lowdown on the Ketogenic (Keto for short) diet. We will be by looking at the basics of using food as fuel and examine the science behind the diet's effectiveness. For all you vegans out there, the advice given in this book, especially regarding nutrition and exercise, applies fully to you as well. The only additional item you need to take care of is figuring out are vegan sources of protein and fat. While fat is easily sourced via seeds and oils, protein is tougher. You need not worry though since a list of vegan protein sources along with supplements are provided.

Along the way, we will also look at specific situations and exercise plans you can implement straight away, no matter which fitness level you're at. There will need to be some level of complexity depending on your goals (for example an athlete versus a rank beginner) but this book will walk you through all of it, step by step.

We will also be busting some myths along the way and vegans need not worry, we'll be covering how the Keto diet can fit seamlessly into your lifestyle!

So sit back and enjoy!

# CHAPTER 1:

## THE BASICS OF NUTRITION

Before we dive into the Keto diet, it is essential that you understand some basics about how our bodies burn the food we consume to provide us with energy and why some foods are good for us and some bad. Understanding this information will help you see why the Keto diet works, far more easily. In addition, you will also be able to evaluate the merits and drawbacks of any other diet you might encounter.

In this chapter, we will break down how the composition of the food you eat affects your health and why your mother was right when she told you to finish your veggies when you were a kid. If you've ever been confused about protein, carbohydrates, vitamins, minerals etc and how they function to aid your well being, this chapter will have all the answers for you!

# NUTRITION AND NUTRIENTS

So what is nutrition? After all, no matter which diet we choose, good nutrition is what we're after. While all of us have some idea of what it is, it's better to define it.

The World Health Organization defines nutrition as follows: Nutrition is the intake of food, considered in relation to the body's dietary needs. Good nutrition – an adequate, well-balanced diet combined with regular physical activity – is a cornerstone of good health. Poor nutrition can lead to reduced immunity, increased susceptibility to disease, impaired physical and mental development, and reduced productivity.[1] ("Nutrition", 2019).

Now that that's out of the way, we can surmise that nutrition is essentially how we feed ourselves. We can do this in a good or a bad way.

## *Balanced Diets*

A balanced diet, from the definition above, simply refers to eating foods from different food groups as part of our daily food intake.

---

[1] Nutrition. 2019. Retrieved from
https://www.who.int/topics/nutrition/en/

[2] Water: How much should you drink everyday?. (2019). Retrieved from
https://www.mayoclinic.org/healthy-lifestyle/nutrition-and-healthy-

The different food groups, roughly speaking, are:

- Vegetables

- Meats

- Grains

- Fruits

- Dairy

Of course, lifestyle choices do affect our ability to follow this advice. This is where it's important to remember how resilient our bodies are. If you're vegan and choose to forego items 2 and 5, this doesn't mean you're condemning yourself to malnutrition. While your nutrition might not be at its most optimum state, this is hardly something to fuss over.

What is far more important to understand is that a balanced diet is recommended because each food group is abundant in a different type of nutrient. Nutrients are what make up all the food we consume. Thus, whether you eat different food groups in a balanced manner or not, what you should be doing is getting a good mix of nutrients in your diet.

## *Nutrients*

There are six major forms of nutrients. They can be listed as:

Carbohydrates: Also called Carbs

- Proteins

- Fats

- Vitamins

- Minerals

- Water

Before everything else, we need to acknowledge that the most important nutrient is water. Our bodies are 60% water and our brains are composed of 70% water. Simply put, without clean, drinkable water, we simply will not survive. No matter which diet you decide to adopt, drinking adequate water is essential. The Mayo Clinic recommends 3.7 liters of water per day for adult men and 2.7 liters per day for adult women [2]**("WATER: HOW MUCH SHOULD YOU DRINK EVERY DAY?" 2019).**

---

[2] Water: How much should you drink everyday?. (2019). Retrieved from https://www.mayoclinic.org/healthy-lifestyle/nutrition-and-healthy-eating/in-depth/water/art-20044256

EACH OF THE ABOVE NUTRIENTS HAS A CERTAIN CALORIC PROFILE, THAT IS, THEY PROVIDE DIFFERENT AMOUNTS OF ENERGY TO OUR BODIES WHEN BURNED. PROTEINS, CARBS AND FATS PROVIDE THE LARGE MAJORITY OF ENERGY WHEN BURNED. VITAMINS AND MINERALS ARE RESPONSIBLE FOR OTHER FUNCTIONS WHILE PROVIDING TRACE AMOUNTS OF ENERGY. THEY ARE RESPONSIBLE FOR A NUMBER OF THINGS SUCH AS BONE HEALTH, IMMUNE SYSTEM HEALTH AND REPAIRING CELLULAR DAMAGE.

WHEN IT COMES TO UNDERSTANDING WEIGHT LOSS AND EVALUATING THE MERITS OF A NEW DIET, OUR MAIN FOCUS RESTS ON PROTEINS, FATS AND CARBS. LET US NOW TAKE A CLOSER LOOK AT EACH OF THESE NUTRIENTS.

### Protein

Proteins are the building blocks of our bodies. They are what help build muscle and tissue. Our bodies convert external proteins into internal ones, like enzymes, and this is how our muscles are maintained and built.

Proteins themselves are made of amino acids, of which there are multiple types. Without going into great detail, animal protein contains a denser distribution of amino acids than plant protein. In other words, if you eat meat, you're likelier to receive your entire amino acid intake in fewer meals as opposed to eating only plants or plant-based food.

Vegans need to eat a wider variety of food to achieve their protein needs. No matter which diet you choose to follow, it is essential you meet your daily protein requirement. Given their function in maintaining muscle, this point should be self-explanatory. The amount of proteins you need to consume daily depends on your lifestyle goals and this will be explored later in this book.

## *Carbohydrates*

Carbs are one of our primary sources of energy. While they do have other essential functions, their main purpose is to provide us with energy to go about our day. Chemically speaking, carbs are simple sugars and starches, which when broken down, turn into glucose which feeds our energy needs.

If you've been paying even a little attention to food-related literature, you will be aware of how bad sugars are supposed to be for you. Now, it is important to realize that naturally occurring sugars, such as those in carbs, are not bad for you. In fact, sugar in appropriate quantities is a part of a balanced diet and you should not be striving to avoid "all" sugar.

If this is confusing, don't worry, we'll cover all this in a later chapter. For now, it is important for you to understand that carbs contain sugar AND, IN THIS FORM, sugar is not bad for you but is essential for healthy body functions.

## Fat

The technically correct scientific term for fat is "lipids" but for simplicity's sake, we will be referring to them as fat or fats. Again, thanks to the influence of popular literature, it is important to note right at the outset: Fat does not make you fat. Neither is fat the only thing that causes you to put on weight. This is an especially relevant point if you are to follow the Keto diet.

Fats also have the same function as carbs in that they are a fuel source, primarily. Fats come in two varieties, saturated and unsaturated. Unsaturated fats, such as coconut and olive oil, are good for you in the right quantities but saturated fats are a bit more controversial.

Thus far, nutritionists agree that saturated fat in excess quantities is harmful but some level of saturated fats are necessary for a balanced diet. Consumed in excess, saturated fats cause hardening of the arteries, that is when arteries get blocked with fat, and cause heart disease. The advice to avoid red meat originates from this fact. Red meat has high amounts of saturated fat and excess consumption will lead to all sorts of unsavory diseases. However, avoiding it entirely isn't appropriate either.

This principle is true of pretty much all kinds of food (with one notable exception) and this is why a lot of confusion crops up. Most people think of nutrition in an either/or sort of way and unfortunately, our bodies have not evolved with an either/or logic. The truth is, everything needs to consume in the appropriate quantity. As long as you stick to the appropriate levels, things are good for you. Cross these limits and its bad. When it comes to nutrition, too much of a good thing is a very real consequence. It is important you approach any diet plan with this philosophy.

Many diets demonize a particular nutrient or macronutrient, and this is simply lacking in scientific fact. So, the next time you see a blanket statement that says "All fats are bad" or "all carbs are unhealthy," know that they are false.

## ENERGY

We've seen in the previous section how our bodies have three primary sources of energy: Proteins, Carbs and Fat. Proteins are probably the most important of the lot because of their role in maintaining our muscles via amino acids. Carbs and fat form the remainder of our fuel sources.

The next bit to understand is that the energy profile of these three is not equal. In other words, one unit of protein does not generate the same amount of energy as one unit of carbs or 1 unit of fat. The energy released by these nutrients are measured in kilocalories (kcal). While technically not the same, in common reference, a kilocalorie is called a "Calorie". Moving forward, to keep things simple, we will refer to this in the same way. Just remember that when we say Calorie, we're talking about kilocalories for simplicity's sake and to avoid confusion with other sources.

The caloric profile of the three major nutrients is listed in the table below:

| NUTRIENT | CALORIES PER GRAM |
|---|---|
| PROTEINS | 4 |
| CARBOHYDRATES | 4 |
| FATS | 9 |

As you can see, fats are more calorie dense than the other two. In other words, to gain the same number of Calories, you need to eat less fat than carbs or proteins. This is an important building block of the Keto diet.

As we go about our day and consume food, our body keeps burning it and realizing energy, via Calories, as per the table above. If we eat as much food, or Calories, as our body needs during the day, we feel sated and can function at a normal level. If we consume less, we will feel a bit hungry, but this isn't a disaster. There is a healthy limit up to which we can consume less than our required Caloric amount per day. Drop below this limit and your body starts breaking down and when prolonged, this becomes unhealthy and leads to all sorts of unwanted consequences.

Similarly there is a healthy limit above your Caloric needs up to which you can consume excess Calories. Go above this limit and you'll, once again, be damaging yourself. Simply put, eat below the healthy limit and you suffer from malnutrition. Eat above the limit and you suffer from obesity. If there was a way to summarize the process of maintaining a healthy weight, that would be it.

### *Weight Loss and Fat Loss*

Most people, when they pick up a book like this, have the aim of weight loss in their mind. What they should be concerned about instead is fat loss. The best way to think of this is as follows: While all fat loss is weight loss, not all weight loss is fat loss.

To examine why this is the case, we need to look at what happens when we eat too much or too little. Let's tackle the former first.

When you consume an excess of calories, your body after burning off whatever it needs to function for the day, has to decide what to do with the surplus calories. What it usually does is, it stores these excess calories as glycogen. This is to ensure you have a decent reserve of energy in case an emergency arises. Glycogen storage is accompanied by a proportional amount of water storage, usually in a 1:3 ratio.

Once the Glycogen stores are filled, if there are any remaining calories left they get stored as fat. This is the fat which shows up in various parts of our body and when it becomes excessive, causes us to reach for a book like this. This is how eating too much makes you fat. Note that at no point does your body differentiate between a Calorie coming from carbs versus protein versus fat. A Calorie is a Calorie no matter where it comes from.

The above narrative oversimplifies the process but as an introduction, this is all you need to know, unless you wish to become a nutritionist. Let us now look at what happens when you run a deficit, that is, you eat less than what you need.

When this happens, your body has a very simple plan. It burns off its stores with priority given to glycogen first and then fat, failing which it will turn to muscle to meet its energy needs. The reason behind this order is not relevant, again, unless you wish to specialize in nutritional science. Suffice to say that, this mechanism is what has evolved in us and serves us well. The body, in this manner always has backup energy to keep you fueled for a certain period, until you refuel.

Given this prioritization of what to burn first, it becomes an easy task for us to determine the best way to lose fat (since we do not wish to lose muscle). We maintain a caloric deficit (that is, eat less than what we need) and once the glycogen stores are depleted, our fat burns off. Of course, we need to take care to not eat too less or else our muscle gets burned as well in the process.

You see, this is the difference between referring to weight loss versus fat loss. Weight loss includes a number of things. If you drink less water, your weight decreases. You could be at your ideal, healthy "weight" and still be unhealthy. The key thing to remember is that you need to minimize the amount of fat in your body and maximize lean muscle. This is where your exercise and diet play a vital role. If your goal is mere weight loss, then starve yourself for a few days. This is the easiest way to lose"weight". However, think of how much damage you're doing to yourself in the process. This is also why starving yourself, in the long term, is never the answer if you're overweight. Controlled caloric deficits are the way to go.

## Exercise

It is entirely possible to lose fat without exercise. Around 80% of your fat loss is dependent on your diet. Why then, you might wonder, should you exercise? After all, isn't the gym one of the most strenuous places to visit? Most people would love the extra hour or so of sleep they would gain.

Exercise has innumerable benefits for your body and all of these are very well known. From a nutrition perspective though, exercise plays a very important role. It helps build muscle. You see, the greater the amount of muscle you have, the easier it is to burn fat and tougher it is to put fat on. Let's see how this works.

When you eat something your body has the option of choosing how it wishes to use this energy. It could use this energy to fuel you (thereby burning all of it) or it could choose to set it aside as either glycogen or fat. The more muscle you have, the more the food that you consume is redirected to feed those muscles and thus less is left over for storage. Why? Well, given that your strength and conditioning is pretty high, the body reasons you don't need as much as emergency storage.

Think of it this way: In a workplace, the more capable someone is at their job, the less likely it is that you, as a manager, need to worry about providing backup to that person should they fail their task. If your team happens to have someone who isn't pulling their weight though, you need to set aside more resources to help compensate for that lag. Your body reasons much the same way.

This doesn't mean the answer is to simply pack on more muscle until you burst. It's just that you need to consistently exercise and make sure your physical and cardiovascular systems are in a healthy state. Once you do this and eat right, the muscle building takes care of itself and in turn any food you eat builds more muscle and your fat content reduces.

Thus, you see, your body helps you stay lean the more you exercise. If you choose to not exercise, your body doesn't see the need to divert more energy towards helping your muscles since they don't require as much energy and neither are they greater in number. Thus the weight you will lose by eating less and not exercising will be an equal proportion of fat and muscle. The net result is you'll lose weight but strength as well. Aesthetically, you'll look about the same, just weaker. Exercise is extremely important to avoid this.

## *Diet*

While it's all fine to say that you need to eat less than you burn to lose weight, what you eat plays an important role. There is a very real difference between good Calories and bad Calories.

Calories from junk food is a prime example of bad Calories. While, in the short run, you will lose weight by eating less junk food than you need to burn, you will be putting a huge amount of stress on your internal systems thanks to the highly processed, chemically altered nature of these foods. Think of it this way: You can be the healthiest looking person alive but still have organ failure. While this is exaggerating it by a lot, it highlights an important point regarding health: You need to be healthy both inside and the outside.

When choosing a diet, you need to begin with proteins as this is absolutely needed for a healthy lifestyle. Consuming protein will help you build and maintain muscle and the amount you ingest, as mentioned previously, will depend on what your goals are. We'll list the exact numbers later but for now, suffice to say, an athlete will need far more protein than someone who exercises twice a week and has a sedentary job.

Once you've determined this, you then have a choice of either balancing carbs and fat or prioritizing one over the other. All choices have their pros and cons and it is here, finally, we arrive at the point of the Ketogenic diet.

The Keto diet prioritizes fats over carbs for a number of reasons we'll be looking at in the next chapter. Before going there though, you still need to keep in mind that if you overeat on the Keto diet, you will still gain weight. The diet is not a magic bullet and the principle guiding fat loss, that is maintaining a caloric deficit, still applies. You will need to exercise when following this diet as well, needless to say.

So, now that we understand the basic principles, let's dive in and look at the Ketogenic diet and why this is the most effective diet for fat loss.

# CHAPTER 2:

## THE KETOGENIC DIET

The Ketogenic diet is, contrary to popular perception, one of the oldest diets out there. Originally developed in the 1920s as a treatment for children suffering from epilepsy

[1] (Mandal, 2019), the Ketogenic diet eventually went mainstream thanks to the effects people started noticing in body composition, apart from the impact on epilepsy itself.

In this chapter we're going to take a deep look at the science behind all of it and why the diet works as spectacularly as it does. We will also see the different modifications you can make to it to suit your lifestyle.

---

[1] Mandal, A. (2019). History of the Ketogenic Diet. Retrieved from https://www.news-medical.net/health/History-of-the-Ketogenic-Diet.aspx

# PRINCIPLES

The Ketogenic diet emphasizes the importance of fats in the diet over carbs given a predetermined level of protein. This diet is shown to offer a number of health benefits, from reducing obesity and epilepsy to even minimizing the chances of contracting cancer and managing diabetes or Alzheimer's disease.

These claims are not simply conjured out of thin air. Keto has been around as long as it has so it's is one of the most intensely studied and dissected diet out there. These studies are largely responsible for dispensing with the notion that eating fat makes us fat. Let us look at some of the more popular studies to better examine the health effects of Keto.

## *Obesity*

A study conducted in 2003 compared the effects of a low carb diet (Keto) versus a low-fat diet on obesity[2] (Foster et al., 2003). Sixty-three subjects were randomly placed into two groups: one which followed a low-fat diet and another which followed a low carb diet.

---

[2] Foster, G., Wyatt, H., Hill, J., McGuckin, B., Brill, C., & Mohammed, B. et al. (2003). A Randomized Trial of a Low-Carbohydrate Diet for Obesity. *New England Journal Of Medicine, 348*(21), 2082-2090. doi: 10.1056/nejmoa022207

The results are summarized below: (Foster et al., 2003)

*In the analysis in which baseline values were carried forward in the case of missing values, the group on the low-carbohydrate diet had lost significantly more weight than the group on the conventional diet at 3 months (P=0.001) and 6 months (P=0.02), but the difference in weight loss was not statistically significant at 12 months.*

In other words, at the 6-month mark, the results clearly showed the subjects on the low carb diet had lost more weight than the other group. However, attrition is high, the study was inconclusive over a period of 12 months. Additionally, the low carb group had greater improvement in triglycerides and HDL.

The efficacy of a low carb diet was studied on healthy women as well to prove that such a diet isn't meant only for those suffering from physical ailments.[3](Brehm, Seeley, Daniels & D'Alessio, 2003). This study tracked 53 healthy but moderately obese women over a period of 6 months. Subjects were randomized into either a low carb diet group or a low-fat diet group.

---

[3] Brehm, B., Seeley, R., Daniels, S., & D'Alessio, D. (2003). A Randomized Trial Comparing a Very Low Carbohydrate Diet and a Calorie-Restricted Low Fat Diet on Body Weight and Cardiovascular Risk Factors in Healthy Women. *The Journal Of Clinical Endocrinology & Metabolism, 88*(4), 1617-1623. doi: 10.1210/jc.2002-021480

The results were just as conclusive and statistically significant as the previous study. The subjects in the low carb group lost, on average, 19 lbs while the women in the other group lost, on average, 8.6 lbs overall. Also, once again, the triglycerides and HDL levels were found to be better in the low carb group. In conclusion, the authors had this to say:

*Based on these data, a very low carbohydrate diet is more effective than a low-fat diet for short-term weight loss and, over 6 months, is not associated with deleterious effects on important cardiovascular risk factors in healthy women*

### Diabetes

A study in 2006 aimed to observe the effects of low carb, restricted diet on patients suffering from Type 2 diabetes. 102 patients were randomized into two groups, again, one following a low fat and the other following a low carb diet plan for a period of 6 months[64](Daly et al., 2006).

The results of this study speak for themselves:[6](Daly et al., 2006)

---

[4] Daly, M., Paisey, R., Paisey, R., Millward, B., Eccles, C., & Williams, K. et al. (2006). Short-term effects of severe dietary carbohydrate-restriction advice in Type 2 diabetes-a randomized controlled trial. *Diabetic Medicine, 23*(1), 15-20. doi: 10.1111/j.1464-5491.2005.01760.x

*Weight loss was greater in the low-carbohydrate (LC) group (−3.55 ± 0.63, mean ± sem) vs. −0.92 ± 0.40 kg, P = 0.001) and cholesterol : high-density lipoprotein (HDL) ratio improved (−0.48 ± 0.11 vs. −0.10 ± 0.10, P = 0.01). However, relative saturated fat intake was greater (13.9 ± 0.71 vs. 11.0 ± 0.47% of dietary intake, P < 0.001), although absolute intakes were moderate.*

## Alzheimer's

A 2006 study found significant evidence that the ketogenic diet does have effects on our brain's neural structure and that this may help reduce the debilitating effect of diseases where cellular level changes affect healthy functioning adversely[5] (Gasior et al., 2006).

The conclusions of this study were significant: (Gasior et al., 2006)

*It has long been recognized that the ketogenic diet is associated with increased circulating levels of ketone bodies, which represent a more efficient fuel in the brain, and there may also be increased numbers of brain mitochondria. It is plausible that the enhanced energy*

---

[5] Gasior, M., Rogawski, M.A., & Hartman, A. L. (2006). Neuroprotective and disease-modifying effects of the ketogenic diet. *Behavioural Pharmacology*, 17(5-6), 431-9.

*production capacity resulting from these effects would confer neurons with greater ability to resist metabolic challenges......*

*Although each of the aforementioned alternatives is still early in development, the idea of developing the ketogenic diet in a 'pill' is very attractive and may be approachable.*

## Brain Cancer

A 2007 study indicated the effectiveness of the Keto diet as an alternative option for malignant brain cancer. While, obviously, not a cure for the disease, the reduction in tumor growth was statistically significant [6](Zhou et al., 2007).

Below are the results observed in the study:(Zhou et al., 2007)

*KetoCal administered in restricted amounts significantly decreased the intracerebral growth of the CT-2A and U87-MG tumors by about 65% and 35%, respectively, and significantly enhanced health and survival relative to that of the control groups receiving the standard low fat/high carbohydrate diet. The restricted KetoCal diet reduced*

---

[6] Zhou, W., Mukherjee, P., Kiebish, M. A., Markis, W. T., Mantis, J. G., & Seyfried, T. N. (2007). The calorically restricted ketogenic diet, effective alternative therapy for malignant brain cancer. Nutrition & Metabolism, 4, 5. doi:10.1186/1743-7075-4-5

*plasma glucose levels while elevating plasma ketone body (beta-hydroxybutyrate) levels. Tumor microvessel density was less in the calorically restricted KetoCal groups than in the calorically unrestricted control groups. Moreover, gene expression for the mitochondrial enzymes, beta-hydroxybutyrate dehydrogenase and succinyl-CoA: 3-ketoacid CoA transferase, was lower in the tumors than in the contralateral normal brain suggesting that these brain tumors have reduced ability to metabolize ketone bodies for energy.*

*The conclusion of this study was that due to the tumor's growth being dependent on glucose, a caloric restriction combined with a high-fat diet slowed the growth of the tumors and that the diet could function as an alternative therapy* [7] *(Zhou et al., 2007)*

## Acne

Yes, even common acne was found to be minimized greatly when following the ketogenic diet. While this study wasn't as conclusive as possible, the results were definitely significant [8] (Paoli et al., 2012).

---

[7] Zhou, W., Mukherjee, P., Kiebish, M. A., Markis, W. T., Mantis, J. G., & Seyfried, T. N. (2007). The calorically restricted ketogenic diet, effective alternative therapy for malignant brain cancer. *Nutrition & Metabolism, 4,* 5. doi:10.1186/1743-7075-4-5

[8] Paoli, A., Grimaldi, K., Toniolo, L., Canato, M., Bianco, A., & Fratter, A.

As must be obvious by now, the keto diet is highly effective in not just losing weight but also in mitigating the debilitating effects of many diseases. The journal articles cited here are just the tip of the iceberg when it comes to the number of studies performed on the diet.

We've already seen how the ketogenic diet is a low carb, high-fat diet. Let's now take a closer look at how it works physically and why it is as effective as it is.

# KETOSIS

This section could have also been named "the secret of Ketogenic diets". Ketosis is why you will lose weight when following this diet. What is Ketosis though and how is it induced? Why is it induced only on a high-fat diet? How does it work? We'll examine the answers in the following sections.

### What is it?

Ketosis is a normal bodily function wherein the body starts burning fat instead of glucose in order to produce energy. As we saw earlier, glucose is the body's primary fuel source and the first in the order of priority when it comes to burning in order to produce energy.

(2012). Nutrition and Acne: Therapeutic Potential of Ketogenic Diets. *Skin Pharmacology And Physiology*, 25(3), 111-117. doi: 10.1159/000336404

When there is a lack of glucose, the body needs an alternate fuel source and fat provides it. As fat is burned, there is a rise of acids called Ketones and their presence in the bloodstream is an indication that the body is burning fat instead of glucose. Ketones are excreted via urine and are a natural by-product of ketosis.

## Safety

Ketosis, if induced, is a fully normal bodily process and you have nothing to fear from it. Excessive levels of it, however, point to issues with the body's ability to produce and use insulin and is an indicator of diabetes.

Indeed, in patients suffering from type 1 diabetes, extreme ketosis is more likely to develop. Ketosis can be safely induced by following a low carb diet. Carbs are a primary source of glucose, given that they are sugars as we saw previously, and once you restrict them, the body is forced to burn fat instead.

Again, this does not mean you starve yourself. Fasting for a day is fine and is an ancient method to induce ketosis in the body but prolonging this state of affairs in unhealthy. This is why it is essential you substitute the Calories lost due to the carb restriction with calories from fats while maintaining an appropriate protein level in your diet.

### *Ketosis and Ketoacidosis*

Ketosis should not be confused with Ketoacidosis which is an extreme condition of ketosis. As ketone levels go beyond safe parameters in the bloodstream, the blood becomes highly acidified and this is a serious medical condition which requires emergency intervention.

This phenomenon is usually observed in people suffering from Type 1 diabetes. While there are instances of it occurring in people with Type 2 diabetes, it is very rare. Now, if you suffer from diabetes, you might be wondering if the Ketogenic diet is safe for you?

### *Effect on Diabetes*

As we saw from the medical studies in the previous section, the keto diet is perfectly safe for patients with Type 2 diabetes. People suffering from Type 1 diabetes will need to consult their doctor on the best course of action to take.

Due to the diabetic condition, where the body does not process insulin effectively, being as it is, doctors often prescribe a low carb diet for patients in order to prevent blood sugar levels from spiking. Having said that, Type 2 diabetes patients need to constantly monitor the ketone level within their bloodstream due to the danger of ketoacidosis.

Ketones do show up in the urine but the best way to measure their level is via a blood test. There are a number of self-testing kits available which do the job excellently. Healthy and desired levels of ketones in the blood amount to 0.5-3 mmol/L. If you wish to measure them via your urine then indicator strips will do the job.

Any person following the keto diet can choose to track their ketone levels to determine whether they are in ketosis or not. There are some other symptoms as well as we shall see next.

### Other Symptoms of Ketosis

Bad breath: Higher levels of ketones mean greater levels of acetone which gives your breath a distinctly fruity flavor. You might need to brush multiple times a day or use sugar-free gum to combat this.

Fast Weight Loss: After initially adopting the keto diet, depending on how much weight you need to lose, you will see a drastic drop in your weight. This is not fat reduction but simply water weight being shed. Remember, in the previous chapter, we saw how water needs to be stored as glucose levels increase? Well, if glucose levels decrease there's no need for excess water so your body gets rid of it.

Decreased energy initially: If you've never had a low carb diet before, adjusting to it takes time. During this time, your body, which is used to burning high amounts of glucose to fuel you, is still looking for glucose simply because it is used to it. Once it figures out there's no glucose it starts to burn fat instead and this is when your energy levels rise. Most dieters report this "keto fog" lasting a week at most. Switching diets over the weekend is a good idea in order to combat this.

Less hunger pangs: On the keto diet, you will see that your hunger isn't as ferocious as it usually is. While the exact reason for this is not known, many dieters have reported this event for it to be statistically significant. Dieticians think this might be the ketones changing the way our brains process hunger.

Changing bowel movements: Constipation and diarrhea are side effects when beginning the keto diet. Due to the reduced number of carbs, and the fiber they provide, your bowel movements usually suffer. This can be mitigated by eating lots of leafy greens or taking a fiber supplement. Getting the amount right takes some trial and error and it is in this period when you might suffer from diarrhea due to taking too much fiber.

So as you can see there are a number of ways to tell if you're in ketosis or not. Getting into ketosis is what the keto diet is all about and it pays to track your state when adopting the diet for the first time.

# KETOGENIC FOODS

So now that we've looked at the science behind the keto diet, understood ketosis and its importance and are up to speed with the basics of nutrition, it's time to finally dig into what to eat when following the ketogenic diet. This section will list everything you should eat and what you should avoid. Vegans will also find plenty of options here so if you are one, you need not worry!

Right off the bat, you need to understand that all chemically-processed foods should be avoided like the plague. This is not a ketogenic diet rule as much as a common sense rule. Highly processed foods contain chemicals which cause harm and you need to avoid these foods. Examples include TV dinners, frozen pizza, fast food, sugary soft drinks and other chemically processed food. A good rule of thumb is to have whole foods as much as possible. For example, cheese is a processed food but a lot of cheese isn't chemically or artificially processed.

Foods labeled "diet" or "low fat" should be avoided as well since more often than not they are chemically altered. Any meat that has had hormones injected into it, needless to say, does not fit the bill. Eating organic as much as possible is the best way forward. This isn't always practical so at the very least, avoid the overly sugary and obviously chemically processed foods for now.

Let's now look at what you should eat on the ketogenic diet.

## Meat

Meat lovers rejoice! All kinds of meat, red, white, steak, chicken and turkey is perfectly compatible with the keto diet. Protein plays an important role in the diet. While the primary aim is to reduce your overall fat levels, a secondary aim is to increase lean body mass or muscle. This in turn helps the primary objective.

Meat is an excellent source of protein. Take care to see that the meat you purchase is of good quality and is hormone-free as much as possible. Also, opt for leaner cuts. Despite the keto diet being a high-fat diet, it isn't a free license for you to load up on fatty cuts. The fats found in meat are usually saturated fats and an excess of this is not healthy.

Opting for chicken breasts instead of thighs, for example, is making a good choice.

## Fatty Fish

Fish make the cut as well on the keto diet. Salmon, tuna and mackerel are examples of excellent, healthy fish you can consume. A cheaper option would be sardines which can be purchased canned or fresh.

When eating fish higher on the food chain like salmon or tuna, you must be careful to avoid mercury poisoning which may occur due to over-consumption. A similar warning applies to smoked salmon. While delicious, the smoking process does cause some chemicals to form which are toxic in large quantities.

### Eggs

Eggs are your go-to protein source. Make sure you eat the yolk as well since the majority of the protein is found there. While the yolk does increase your harmful cholesterol, with regular exercise and a diet which is healthy overall, the harmful effects are greatly reduced to the point of not existing.

Ideally, you should consume omega-3, organic free range eggs but again if this is not an option, try to consume eggs which are as close to organic as possible.

### Butter and Cream

Off all the foods on the keto diet, these are the ones people have the most trouble consuming. Years of conditioning about how fat is bad for you and how it clogs your arteries have lead people to swearing off these completely healthy options.

Moderation is key here and again, choosing the best sourced, organic options is the right decision. Clarified butter (ghee) is also an excellent choice.

## Nuts and Seeds

Almonds, walnuts, chia seeds are excellent sources of healthy fats with relatively low carbs. They are the best option when you feel the need for a snack. Be careful to not overeat though! It's very easy to eat too much and throw your Calorie counts off!

## Oils

Oils are one of the worst offenders when it comes to chemical processing. Extra refined, frying oil, which is almost as clear as water is one of the worst things you can choose to consume.

Instead, choose whole oils like olive oil, coconut oil, almond oil, mustard oil and avocado oil. When purchasing these, make sure they are either virgin or cold pressed. You will find options these days for something called olive pomace oil. This is marketed as olive oil and is far cheaper than regular extra virgin olive oil. Stay away from it though since it is chemically treated and is just a marketing gimmick.

Cooking with these oils does take some getting used to since they tend to smoke at lower temperatures compared to refined oils. Also they do have a stronger taste due to their untarnished nature.

## *Low Carb Vegetables*

On the keto diet you should avoid starchy, high carb vegetables like the following

- Tubers

- Carrots

- Beets

- Corn

- Green Peas

- Parsnips

- Sweet potato

- Pumpkin

- Yams

Instead, low carb options like the ones below

- Onions

- Peppers

- Tomatoes

- Spinach

- Kale

- Asparagus

- Broccoli

- Salad Greens

- Cucumber

While technically a fruit, the avocado belongs here. If the keto diet had to have a face, it would have to be the avocado's. Have it raw, as guacamole or as part of a salad, this fatty fruit has it all.

### Miscellaneous

Condiments are a sneaky way to inadvertently cheat on the keto diet. Ketchup, mustard and the like are permissible as is salt and pepper. The thing you want to look out for is the sugar content of these condiments.

So a full fat ranch dressing might sound keto friendly but a store-bought item will almost invariably have a high amount of sugar in it. This is unlikely to be naturally-occurring sugar so stay away from it.

Artificial sweeteners can be used such as stevia, xylitol and sorbitol. While not a great idea, having some occasionally is perfectly fine. Coffee and tea are perfectly fine as long as they are consumed black and preferably unsweetened. Adding dairy to it will improve the keto-friendliness of it.

If you're a chocolate lover, dark chocolate is a wonderful option. Make sure to consume something with more than 80% cocoa though and organic if possible.

This concludes the list of permissible things to eat. As you can see there are many options and there's no real need to restrict yourself in any way. The key thing to keep in mind is that moderation in everything is key. Yes, you can consume cream and butter but this does not give you the license to down a full tub of it. Excess of anything is harmful and you need to maintain a caloric deficit, even on the keto diet, to lose fat.

Vegans might be panicking at this point because there don't seem to be many protein sources available. Indeed, meat is out of the question and the usual vegan protein sources like chickpeas and legumes are not compatible. There is a solution for this.

Among whole food, your protein choices are low to be honest. The best, perhaps only, keto sources of protein are:

- Seitan

- Tempeh

- Tofu

That's not much of a list. The best thing to do is to supplement using a vegan protein powder. Remember that going vegan is a great choice but you do need to put in some work to get the benefits. Do not give in to the temptation to consume less protein since it is absolutely essential you eat enough depending on your lifestyle goals.

Let us now look at the foods you ought to avoid on the keto diet.

# FOODS TO AVOID

While we're clear on the fact that processed foods ought to be avoided, it still bears fruit to run through the list of foods you should not be eating. There will be some foods which you are used to eating which will not make the cut. Some of these might surprise you.

### *Sugary Foods*

Sodas, fruit juices, ice cream, candy, chocolate cake, unless they happen to be keto versions, all fall under this category. This seems like a lot to give up, especially if you have a sweet tooth. Dark chocolate is the only substitute you have for this category and with discipline, you will find that you don't miss these foods anymore.

## Grains

All grains like rice, wheat, barley, buckwheat and bulgur are to be avoided. You can substitute this with high protein grains like quinoa but you need to be aware of the amount of carbs you're consuming.

Fruits contain a high amount of naturally occurring sugar. While they are not unhealthy per se, given the presence of sugar, they do tend to increase the amount of glucose produced upon consumption. This, of course, interrupts the process of ketosis.

You can consume berries like strawberries, blueberries and raspberries.

## Beans and Legumes

Legumes and beans are a great vegan source of protein but given the carb ratio in them, they are not suitable for a ketogenic diet. As detailed above though, there are ways to substitute for them successfully.

## Tubers

Generally speaking, any starchy or root vegetable is not suited for the keto diet. So potatoes, sweet potatoes, turnips, beets, carrots and the vegetables listed in the list of starchy foods are out.

You can consume veggies like leafy greens, tomatoes, onions, cauliflower, cabbage, peppers, broccoli, kale etc.

## *Alcohol*

This one should go without saying but alcohol should be minimized on the keto diet. Sticking to clear liquors which are have an alcohol content of over 40% will not throw you out of ketosis. Examples of this are vodka, whiskey, gin and scotch. The real issue with alcohol is the decreased consciousness and hunger pangs it brings and after a few drinks you might not be so inclined to stay disciplined when faced with a pizza. Also, almost all commercially available alcohol contains either added sugar or corn syrup. While the quantities are not large, much like saturated fat as explained previously, minimizing alcohol is the best way forward.

This list of foods to avoid tends to produce an adverse reaction. After all, a non-sugar, non-alcohol consuming existence does tend to be a bit boring. Well, fear not. As we'll see in the chapter dealing with meal plan design, there is a way to satisfy your cravings and still meet your goals.

As always, the message to keep in mind is moderation in everything. Now that we've finished with our in-depth look at the basics of the keto diet, let's now look at the different types of keto diets you can adapt based on your lifestyle goals.

# CHAPTER 3:

## TYPES OF KETOGENIC DIETS

Your lifestyle goals largely dictate your diet and exercise plan. It isn't enough to simply say "I want to lose fat". You also need to define what activity level you wish to carry out to achieve your goals.

You see, losing fat isn't just for the obese. You can be a perfectly healthy individual but wish to shed a few pounds of fat. The keto diet will help you do this in a healthy and controlled manner. Depending on your activity level, there are four options you could follow:

- The Standard Ketogenic Diet

- The High Protein Ketogenic Diet

- The Cyclical Ketogenic Diet

- The Targeted Ketogenic Diet

We'll go over them one by one starting with the standard diet. Before we dive in though, please keep in mind, when starting out it is a good idea to keep track of your macros. This means, you track the carbs, fat and protein you're consuming. Once you're following the diet for a few weeks, you will gain an idea of roughly how much you're eating and whether this is correct or not. Also, all these diet principles apply equally to vegans so there's no additional advice or actions you need to take.

## THE STANDARD KETOGENIC DIET

This is the boilerplate diet that fits almost everyone out there. This diet follows the rules laid out in the previous chapter, that is, low carbs and high fat. Whether you choose to follow this diet or not depends on your activity level.

### *Activity Level and Macros*

For those who perform moderately intense activities like cycling, jogging, playing sports as recreation 2-3 times per week or even train in the gym 3-4 times per week, the standard diet (SKD) is ideal.

Now, estimating your activity level is a tricky thing. If you're a beginner you will almost always overestimate this. If you tend to perform high-intensity exercises (which we will cover later in detail), the standard diet isn't for you. This diet is excellent for those looking to shed a few pounds of fat and generally get into good shape.

The SKD is ideal if your exercise consists mostly of aerobic exercise like running, biking and other activities which involve minimal weight training. When starting off, you will experience a performance dip. The reason for this is similar to why you will experience the keto "fog" when starting out: your body just hasn't adjusted as yet.

Now on the SKD, you want to maintain the following macro ratio (macro refers to macronutrients, that is, proteins, carbs and fat). You need to eat at least 0.7-0.8 grams of protein for every pound of body weight. Next, you need to eat a maximum of 30 grams of carbs. The rest of your Calories should come from fat. Let's look at an example to see how this calculation plays out. First let's list our assumptions:

*Weight in pounds= 180*

*Target caloric intake= 2200 kcal*

Now let's assume we decide to eat 0.8 grams of protein per pound of body weight per day. Using the table in the first chapter (where the Calories per gram for the macros was listed), we can calculate the following:

*Amount of protein eaten in grams= 180\*0.8= 144 grams*

*Calories from protein= 144\*4= 576 kcal*

Next, we know the amount of carbs we're restricting ourselves to. It is recommended to begin with 30g and then reduce after a month or so, once you feel comfortable.

*Amount of carbs eaten in grams= 30*

*Calories from carbs (using the same table)= 30\*4=120 kcal*

*Total calories from protein and carbs= 576+120= 696 kcal*

Given our caloric intake target of 2200 kcal, we now can see that we need to provide 1504 kcal from fat. (points 2-7)

Referring to the same table in chapter 1, we know that each gram of fat yields 9 kcal. So to generate 1504 kcal we need to eat:

*Grams of fat to consume per day= 1504/9= 167 g*

Thus, our final macros are the following: 144g protein, 30g carbs and 167 g fat for a total of 2200 kcal per day.

This is how straightforward it is to calculate your macros. As you can see, once you get past the confusion and just stick to the basics, knowing what to eat and how much becomes a very simple task. It is these calculations upon which you will base your meals and diet plans.

## Caloric Deficit

Now you might be wondering how we arrived at the figure of 2200 kcal in the first place? In other words, how do you determine how many Calories you need to eat in the first place? The answer lies in understanding a term called the BMR or Basal Metabolic Rate.

The BMR is the measure of how much energy a person expends on a given day given their activity level. This number is expressed in kcal and depends on the person's sex, age, height, weight and activity level. The activity level is the only wild card in all of this so it's better to underestimate how active you are when you're starting off.

There are a number of calculators online where you simply input these numbers and you receive your BMR. Now this number is the amount of calories you need to eat to *maintain* your current physical state. After all this is the amount of energy you expend daily. So if you eat this amount, you will maintain. This caloric level is called the *maintenance level* (clever, isn't it?).

If you wish to lose fat, you need to maintain a healthy caloric deficit as previously explained. So how much of a deficit is healthy? Roughly speaking, a 500 kcal deficit is considered healthy. The reason is this: over a 7 day period, maintaining a 500 kcal deficit results in an overall deficit of 500*7= 3500 kcal. This is how much you need to shed one pound of body fat. So at this rate, you will be shedding one pound per week and 4 pounds per month and so on.

Losing weight at a rate greater than this is not recommended for beginners. If you're experienced, you probably don't need to read all of this to begin with.

This is how you safely lose weight in a healthy manner and ensure you are not losing any muscle. We will discuss tracking progress and gains in a later chapter. For now, remember this simple process:

Calculate BMR (via online calculators)

Subtract 500 kcal from it. This is how much you need to eat per day

Eat 0.8 grams of protein per pound of body weight per day. Calculate kcal from protein

Eat 30 grams of carbs per day. Calculate kcal from carbs

Add numbers in steps 2 and 3. Subtract this sum from the number in step 2.

Divide the resulting number by 9 to determine grams of fat you need to eat per day.

Track all metrics and adjust as required (discussed in later chapters)

The only thing left to do is determine your food list and your exercise plan. These will be covered in chapters ahead so don't worry. The aim here is to slowly build your knowledge and comfort level as opposed to overloading you with information.

Next, let us look at the high protein keto diet (HPKD).

## THE HIGH PROTEIN KETOGENIC DIET

The high protein diet is quite similar to the SKD except for one thing. The amount of protein you'll be eating is increased. It is very important to understand when to use this diet and its aims. It all starts with delving into why you would even want to increase protein in the first place.

### *Protein and Muscle*

As we saw in the first chapter where we covered the basics of nutrition, proteins are the building blocks of our muscles. Our muscles are literally made of amino acids which is the same stuff proteins are made of. Hence, the more protein you consume, the more food your muscles have. Right?

Well, not exactly. Our bodies aren't that easy to manipulate. The thing with protein is that beyond a certain amount, our bodies just can't process them anymore as intended and these excess proteins get converted into fat. Recall that our bodies have a priority list when it comes to converting food into either muscle or fat once it has converted food into whatever we need for energy.

If we've already fed our muscles, via a high amount of protein, there is no need to convert it into even more muscle and hence, the excess protein gets converted into fat. The trouble doesn't end there though.

## *Risks*

Excess protein poses many health risks. The nitrogen prevalent in amino acids poses an especial risk to your liver. A 2002 study conducted amongst active athletes found a more concentrated urine as well as increased levels of blood urea nitrogen, which is a measure of kidney function[1](Cronkleton & Sullivan, 2019).

Other risks include weight gain, constipation, diarrhea and a deficit of calcium. A side effect of this is also an increased risk of cancer, thanks to the copious amounts of meat one will presumably eat when following a very high protein diet.

So, while the bro in your gym might preach protein, remember that like everything else, balance is essential.

---

[1] Cronkleton, E., & Sullivan, D. (2019). What Happens If You Eat Too Much Protein?. Retrieved from https://www.healthline.com/health/too-much-protein#recommended-daily-protein

## Balance

So, what is the healthy level of protein consumption? In adult males, this is a maximum of 1.5 grams per pound of body weight and in women it is 1.2 grams per pound of body weight. Anything above this is considered excessive.

When following the keto diet, given its emphasis on fat, if the additional calories you will consume from protein put you over your caloric limit, remove the excess by limiting the amount of carbs you eat, not fat.

## Objective

This brings us back to our original point as to why you would want to eat a higher level of protein to begin with? Given that it helps build muscle, the answer is simple: If you wish to build more muscle, you increase the amount of protein you eat every day.

Now, if you want to build muscle, that is increase your body weight via more muscle, you cannot do this while maintaining a caloric deficit. Your body needs additional fuel to build things and it stands to reason it can't do anything if it doesn't have this excess fuel.

Thus, if your goal is solely to cut fat, an HPKD is not your solution. You need to either follow the SKD or one of the other two variations. If you're a beginner looking to add more muscle, the HPKD is a great choice since its straight forward like the SKD. The only difference is you maintain a caloric excess instead of a deficit.

### Exercise and Excess

The amount of caloric excess you will need to maintain is 500 kcal. Much like how we saw with the SKD, this will result in your gaining 1 lb of muscle in body weight per week. The calculation of your macros is exactly the same as with the SKD.

This time instead of using 0.8 grams per pound of body weight, you use 1.2 to 1.5 grams of protein and calculate those calories. The amount of carbs remain the same and the remaining amount is sourced from fat.

Your exercise regimen plays an important role in building muscle. Following a plan of just cardiovascular exercises like cycling or aerobics will not build you muscle beyond a certain point. You will need to hit the weight room and follow a structured plan based on progressive overloading.

If that sounds like Greek to you, don't worry we'll cover all this in the chapters on building an exercise plan.

## *Tracking*

With the HPKD, tracking is of even greater importance than the SKD. This is because with this diet plan, we're trying to achieve two objectives as opposed to just one. We're trying to build muscle while minimizing fat gain (as opposed to just losing fat with the SKD).

We'll cover this in greater detail later but for now keep in mind that you will have to track not just your food intake but also your exercise performance. You will initially suffer a dip in performance of course but once your body adapts, you should see an increase in strength as time progresses.

Generally, while looking to build muscle, cardio is not recommended since this inhibits muscle growth but rather than eliminate it completely, it is a good idea to merely minimize it. So if you usually do 30 minutes of cardio, reduce it to 10 and so on. HIIT or high-intensity cardio is not recommended on this diet, not because of a lack of performance, but simply because HIIT will burn your muscle along with the fat and this is contrary to your objectives.

Some people, no matter how hard they try, take longer to adapt to the keto diet. If you're one of these people, there is a solution for you. It is the CKD or Cyclical Ketogenic Diet.

# THE CYCLICAL KETOGENIC DIET

As the name suggests, in this variation of the keto diet, you cycle in and out of ketosis. The idea is to get your body used to adapting by forcing it to switch between burning both glucose and fat as fuel.

This is also ideal for those who wish to test the waters when it comes to keto and are perhaps not ready to fully immerse themselves as yet. Now this is a good time to point out that the CKD is actually the most versatile of the ketogenic diet variations in that both beginners and more advanced dieters can implement this.

In the CKD, you will be consuming a high fat, low carb diet for five days of the week and for two days, you will switch to a moderate carb, moderate fat diet, that is, a normal diet. The idea is to replenish your glycogen stores in order to fuel your workouts or physical activities for the following week. If you're a beginner or someone who just isn't able to adapt to the SKD immediately or even after a week, this cycling helps ease you into the SKD gradually.

Given that these are two very different objectives, its well worth it to break down how the diet should work for both scenarios.

## *Gradual Easing*

When starting out on the keto diet, if you don't perform and don't plan on performing any strenuous physical activity, the SKD is your best option. The drawback with this is the SKD adopts a sink or swim approach. If you're choosing to adopt the keto diet over a weekend, it might go like this: On Thursday, you have a regular amount of carbs. On Friday, all of a sudden, you're eating next to no carbs and huge amounts of fat.

Mentally and physically this is quite a change to make. Our bodies and minds are extremely resilient so you will be able to handle it without too many issues beyond the "fog" phase. For some though, this fog lasts longer or for whatever reason, they just take longer to adapt to the food they'll be eating now.

For example someone who has been consuming grains and legumes for their meals for over 20 years, suddenly giving this up will not be easy. They will feel the need to have something filling in their meals, that is, something that replicates the full feeling grains give them post meal times. If such people choose to eat salads, then there are two issues: 1) Salads don't give that full feeling and 2) They might 32not be able to digest raw vegetables easily leading to digestive issues.

For such people, CKD makes sense since it allows them to mentally and physically ease into the diet.

## Goals

The first week after trying and failing to adopt the SKD, you could start the CKD. It is a good idea to keep your carb consuming days back to back, preferably towards the end of the week. You can have one of these days coincide with your cheat day, a concept we'll talk about when we look at the process of designing a meal plan. Remember, throughout all of this, you will be maintaining a caloric deficit.

During the two days, you will be consuming carbs, aim for the following when calculating your macros.

Keep the protein level the same as you usually would

Aim to eat 20% of your Calories from fat

That's all there is to it. So, you will need to calculate your macros for these two days and figure out what you need to eat in what quantity. The period after you eat your carbs is more important when it comes to ensuring you progress towards your goals. You should aim to enter ketosis as soon as possible once you've finished your carb loading days.

The best way to do this is on the day following your second carb day, eat almost no carbs or 10g at the most. This forces your body to adapt and start burning fat for fuel. It also hastens the onset of ketosis and gets your body used to the fact that it needs to adapt fast and change the way it derives fuel.

Ideally, you don't want to stretch this cyclical period out to more than a month. It's easy to get comfortable doing this but remember the aim is to eventually move onto the SKD. Always keep this in mind when following the CKD.

Now, if you're someone who's more experienced with dieting and are used to performing high-intensity exercises, the CKD works for you as well. Let's see how.

Performance Oriented CKD

The idea of the carb loading that occurs as a part of CKD is to replenish your glycogen stores to fuel your workouts. This way you can continue to make gains in the gym while cutting fat and getting all the benefits of the keto diet. The other advantage of the CKD is that your body is not being deprived of carbs for long periods, as it would be with the SKD, and this assists your recovery and overall health.

When designing the schedule, you don't need to over think the times your carb loading days need to occur. The usual practice is to have them back to back on your weekly workout schedule. If you workout alternate days, you can have the first day on a workout day and second on a rest day or the other way around. The only scenarios to avoid are to have both days fall on rest days or have the day following the second day be a rest day.

This way you get the full benefit of carbs for muscle building and the benefits of the SKD during the remaining days. There are some things you will need to take into consideration though.

### Macro Ratios

On your first loading day, your macro ratio should be 70% carbs, 20% proteins, and 10% fats. This, as you can see, is the exact opposite of the SKD. On the second carb loading day, change your ratio to 60% carbs, 25% proteins and 15% fat. In other words, you eat slightly fewer carbs and a little more protein and fat on the second day.

Opinion is divided as to when the carbs ought to be consumed. Conventional wisdom tells us that carbs are good for muscle growth and naturally, consuming them post workout seems ideal. However, there is also a branch of thought which proposes that carbs post workout may actually be hindering performance. As with all things nutrition, all these highlights is how much we still don't know how our bodies work.

Here's the best way to tackle this: On the first day, eat your carbs pre and post workout in whatever ratio you feel comfortable with. Go with whatever is the easiest and most comfortable for you. On the second day, your priority should be to get back into ketosis as soon as possible. Hence, consume carbs only pre-workout.

## *Which Carbs?*

Not all carbs are created equal. Whether you're executing the CKD as a beginner or as an intermediate, it is essential for you to pick the right type of carbs for your nutrition. As a beginner, it is ideal for you to pick low GI carbs on your loading days. For the intermediates out there, pick a low GI carb on the first day and high GI carbs on the second day.

What is GI some of you might be wondering? Well, GI stands for glycemic index. This index which runs from 0-100 is a measure of the rapidity with which carb is digested and metabolized. Foods which rank high on the GI scale tend to get metabolized faster and result in a spike in blood sugar levels followed by a subsequent drop. Slower burning carbs of lower GI carbs produce a more even distribution and lesser spikes.

While high GI carbs by themselves sound bad, remember this applies for carbs eaten in significant quantities over a period of time. On the keto diet, you're not consuming anywhere near enough. However, to be on the safe side it's better to stick to low GI carbs. Examples of this include sweet potatoes, lentils and soy products.

## Ketosis

You need to aim to get back into ketosis as soon as possible and this begins post workout on your second carb loading day. If you choose to have the second loading day on a rest day, no matter, aim to finish your carbs quota by early evening. Following this, you need to begin the process of hastening ketosis as much as possible.

This begins with a fasted workout the next morning. Ideally, this will be a long HIIT workout or a strength training workout followed by a small HIIT session. Make sure you supplement with BCAA prior to working out or else you will lose muscle. BCAA means BCAA, not protein powder or creatine. You need to fuel your muscles directly and as quickly as possible prior to workout.

Also fasted means no coffee or juice or anything. Just water and fat burner supplement should you need one and you're good to go. This regime forces your body to burn any excess glycogen it might have from the previous two days and to start using fat as fuel, that is, ketosis.

It is also a good idea to reduce the number of carbs you consume on this day to 10 grams to further emphasize the state of ketosis.

## *Goals and Results*

It pays to constantly keep your goals in mind with all this since there is a fair amount of tracking required. With this sort of cycling followed by high-intensity workouts, you will be changing your body composition. Therefore, it doesn't make sense to be in a deficit. Your aim should instead be maintenance. You can experiment with a slight deficit of say 250kcal per day but it might be too strenuous, especially for your post carb loading early morning workout.

Sticking to this religiously will recompose your lean body mass and fat percentage. Due to the cycling occurring, it is a good idea to purchase ketone testing strips, either via blood tests or urine to ensure you're entering ketosis as planned following your loading days.

## *Consistency*

As mentioned previously the keto diet is not a magic bullet. The key is consistency and repeated action. Best results are obtained over a period of at least 90 days. This is when physical changes will be apparent and you'll be able to see them in the mirror.

Ultimately staying disciplined will help you achieve your goals than any diet out there. It will be difficult to stay in a caloric deficit for example for very long but if you remain mentally strong you will see your efforts bear fruit.

The CKD is a versatile option but sometimes, it just becomes a little too cumbersome. Calculating and tacking your different macro levels might seem like too much work for too little payoff. This is where the Targeted Ketogenic Diet or TKD comes in.

## THE TARGETED KETOGENIC DIET

One of the drawbacks with the CKD is that it requires you to step out of ketosis and re-enter. While the body is more than capable of handling this, mentally this does become taxing over longer periods of time. Over and above this, if you have cheat meals as most people do, you will find it difficult to schedule this along with your loading days and with the wrong schedule, you will find yourself out of ketosis quite a lot.

Naturally, if this happens a lot, you won't be receiving the full benefit of switching to a keto diet in the first place. This is where the TKD helps.

## Precise Loading

The TKD functions on the same premise as the CKD, except the carb loading period is squeezed into a window right before your workout. The amount of carbs you eat is also tightly controlled. The idea is that the carbs help fuel your workout and performance and ideally, they glucose from the carbs will be exhausted within that time period, leaving you free to slip back into ketosis right after.

Reality is rarely this clean but the idea works more often than not. Again, the TKD is a diet for someone who performs high-intensity exercises or activities. If you're a beginner looking to lose fat, the SKD is your best bet.

## Timing

To execute the TKD all you need to do is consume carbs around an hour prior to your workout. The amount of carbs consumed should be around 30 grams and not more than this. Also, needless to say, these carbs should be consumed only pre-workout, not post workout.

Your post-workout meal and nutrition are based on regular keto diet principles, that is high fat and low carb. Usually, you will find yourself out of ketosis for a few hours post workout but after that time period, it will restart. If you find yourself out of ketosis for extended periods for whatever reason, work out the next day on an empty stomach, with adequate BCAA supplementation, and you'll find yourself back in ketosis soon.

If this is a regular occurrence, there's something going wrong in your nutrition which bears examining.

### *High and Low GI*

For your pre-workout carb load, you want to be consuming high GI carbs. This is because you need something to fuel you up quickly. A lower GI carb will not give you enough glucose in time for your workout, not to mention delay your ketosis onset.

You should also keep in mind that carb loading is not a license for you to binge and eat all sorts of junk. Very often, there is a mistaken belief that since you'll be burning everything anyway, you could just eat whatever you want. You still have to follow proper nutrition rules, that is, stay away from processed foods or foods high in sugar.

Sugary food and drink will seem like the best option for a pre-workout load since they provide instant energy. The long term effects of processed sugar are damaging though and you ought to stay away from it.

## *Post Workout*

Your post-workout nutrition should follow regular keto diet rules. A protein shake is the best option if you cannot have a heavy meal immediately.

This concludes our look at the different types of keto diets. As you can see there is an option available for everyone, no matter where on the experience scale you fall. The most important thing to remember is that your diet needs to be allied to your activity level.

We'll be looking at the activity levels and the various workout you can fit into them later in the book. For now though, it is important we look at one of the most overlooked areas of dieting: supplementation.

# CHAPTER 4:

# SUPPLEMENTS

Supplements get a bad rep mostly due to ignorance and other commercial factors. Say the word supplement and most people immediately think of steroids. While steroids are a form of supplement, they are far removed from the world of regular supplements. It's a bit like saying all fish in the ocean are like sharks and that you should avoid swimming near all of them.

On the keto diet, it is not strictly necessary for you to supplement. They do help though. For vegans, it is absolutely necessary since there just aren't enough protein options out there. Another reason to supplement is to help fuel your workouts. You see, the best way to lose fat is to work out in a fasted state. Now, as you can imagine, it is pretty difficult to get going on an empty stomach. You simply cannot do this without the help of supplements.

Supplements have come a long way since the early days when almost everything was some sort of steroid. While they are completely safe, you still ought to remember they are called supplements for a reason. They merely assist you in your diet. They are not a diet in and as of themselves. Given the volume of them in the market, it can be difficult to remember this. Whole food is still your best bet to achieve all your nutritional goals.

Let us now look at some of the most useful supplements and some other not so useful ones which are simply a drain on your wallet for all purposes. All of these are vegan friendly and in the case of protein powder, vegan friendly options are available as noted.

## USEFUL SUPPLEMENTS

It is not necessary for you to purchase these supplements, but they are nice to have. The ones which are absolutely necessary for certain people, for example, vegans, will be highlighted clearly.

### *Multivitamins*

These are the most popular supplements taken regularly by people. The reality, however, is that their degree of helpfulness is still not fully clear. While we do know that a deficiency of vitamins is bad for our immune system and that it increases our risk of heart disease and other undesirable conditions, we still don't know whether ingesting them in a pill form is as effective as it ought to be. The consensus is that consuming them via whole food is the best but it is extremely difficult and counterproductive to track vitamin consumption like macros. Hence, everyone seems to agree that doing something is better than nothing so pills are the best option we have as of now.

Some of the most common deficiencies found are for Vitamin D and Vitamin B12. Vitamin D, as most of you may know, is produced via exposure to sunlight. This is an especial problem for people in countries which suffer from extended winters. In such cases, a specialized Vitamin D supplement is recommended along with a general multivitamin.

B12 is often found deficient in vegans and vegetarians since this is found exclusively in animal products. Needless to say, if you're a vegan living in Norway, your first purchase ought to be a multivitamin supplement. If you're over the age of 50, multivitamins are a must for you, whether you're on the keto diet or not.

### Creatine

Creatine is a bit controversial as a supplement. You see, there's no doubt that it does help stimulate muscle growth.

The issue is whether you actually need it if you're able to more than eat whole food. Some studies report the gains to be marginal and some indicate that creatine is often a direct stimulant. One wonders why there's so much confusion around nutrition!

When it comes to the keto diet, supplementing creatine is a choice that depends on your goals. If you're looking to build muscle then adding creatine to your diet is worth it. If you're looking to cut fat or recompose your physique then on a keto diet creatine probably isn't going to make a significant difference. It will have an effect no doubt but since your goal is not to build muscle, it might not be the most effective use of it.

As a beginner, you really don't need creatine. In fact, at this stage, you're better off with a few supplements. This is because, at a beginner's stage, almost anything you do will make a huge difference. Strength gains in the gym will give you a much better physique than creatine ever will. So focus on exercising well and building up your expertise in that regard.

If you're performing high-intensity activities with the goal of building muscle as part of your workout routine then creatine is a perfect choice. Combined with whey protein, creatine will give you major performance gains and will also reduce your need to load on high GI carbs.

## *Omega 3*

Here's a fun fact: Our brain's composition is 40% DHA which is an omega 3 fatty acid. If you aren't eating fatty fish every week, you're one of the many people who are deficient in this. Fish oil is the most well-known supplement for omega 3 with the capsules containing doses of both EPA and DHA, another omega 3 acid.

Recommended intake is 250-500 mg per day. Depending on the size of the capsule, your dosage will vary. This supplement is necessary no matter which diet you follow.

Vegans need not worry, there are readily available plant sources for omega 3. It must be said, however, that plant sources aren't as rich compared to fish and you will have to consume a lot more of them in order to meet your requirement. Chia seeds, flax seeds, walnuts, and hemp seeds are excellent plant-based sources. Flax seeds also double as an excellent fiber supplement which we'll be looking at next, so they are a win-win.

The best way to meet this requirement would be to mix the powder of these seeds into your meals throughout the day as opposed to setting aside a particular time to eat it.

## *Fiber*

On a high protein, high-fat diet, you will suffer from a lack of fiber. There's no getting away from it. One way of increasing the amount of fiber in your diet is to eat a lot of leafy green vegetables like lettuce, cabbage and spinach.

However, you are not a rabbit and there's only so much lettuce you can eat. A fiber supplement is essential to prevent constipation and other nasty surprises. For a change, the vegans have it easier here since the greater amount of plant-based foods their diet has, the overall fiber content will be higher. For meat eaters, any off the shelf fiber supplement will more than do the job, there's no need to get creative with this.

## *Whey and Casein Protein*

Whey and casein protein are both found in milk. However, with dairy being off limits, the best way to supplement this, if needed, is to consume protein powder. You will usually see whey powder and casein powder being sold separately and lots of articles online about how one is better than the other. Let's break this down a little.

The only difference between the two you need to be aware of is that whey is a fast acting protein and casein is a slow acting one. This means whey behaves much like a high GI carb and immediately gives you the boost you need while casein is released slower into the bloodstream. Both have their advantages. Whey gives you an instant performance boost and is excellent as a pre-workout shake. Casein is useful because it provides a steady, sustained stream of protein for your muscles over a longer period, especially relevant if you consume it before going to bed.

If you're vegan, a vegan whey protein powder is absolutely essential, as mentioned previously. Don't try to second guess this and think you can eat more tofu or something, just go buy one. The amount you consume will be dictated by your macro calculations.

For the rest, it really depends on your goals and whether you're comfortable eating more or less whole food. If you're looking to build muscle, then a casein protein powder is a good idea since it will minimize muscle breakdown overnight and aid recovery. If you're trying to lose fat, this is much like creatine and you can take a call either way.

### *BCAA*

Branch chain amino acids or BCAA is something we've touched upon previously when talking about the CKD and TKD. If you're on the SKD you really don't need this. For those on the CKD or TKD, this is absolutely essential for your morning fasted workouts.

Those on the SKD might want to consider this if they wish to workout fasted. This is not something recommended for beginners, even though it results in the fastest fat loss since it takes a lot of mental strength to do this. You won't see too many experienced gym rats training fasted unless they absolutely have to.

There are a lot of recent studies being done recently which are rethinking the way BCAAs work and whether they are useful or not. At this point there haven't been enough conclusions to be statistically significant so for now, we will just rely on the experience of trainers over the years. This is something to watch out for, however.

So to summarize, consuming around 10g BCAA prior to your fasted workout and have a protein shake post workout. You don't really need BCAA if you're not training fasted.

### *Fat Burner*

This is another supplement you need to take only if you're working out fasted. Fat burners don't actually burn fat, they're just branded that way. What they do is they give you a burst of energy which propels you to workout harder than you usually would and thus, burn more Calories.

If you feel especially lethargic in the mornings, then consider supplementing some fat burner. If not, leave it be. A cup of coffee without milk works just as well.

## *Mineral Tablets*

Minerals like zinc, calcium, and magnesium serve major purposes when it comes to your bodily functions. Supplementing them is always a good idea, especially zinc, which will help aid your recovery post workout. The best way of ingesting them, as mentioned previously, is via whole food. As long as you ensure your diet is well balanced and has healthy amounts of leafy greens you will almost certainly be consuming the required quantities of minerals.

In addition, on the keto diet, you will experience a lot of water loss and with that comes a loss of electrolytes like sodium, magnesium, potassium and calcium. You will need to keep track of your water intake and be on the lookout for signs of dehydration like headaches, decreased performance and activity levels.

Your diet should be balanced enough to cover all your needs if you consume food as directed in this book but its recommended you supplement with tablets as well to reduce the risk of deficiencies..

# SUPPLEMENTS YOU DON'T NEED

The market is awash with stuff you don't need unless you're a bodybuilder, and even they only need steroids. So, this list is of stuff you really need not pay any attention to, even if you're looking to build muscle or optimize your workouts. Some of them are actually good but are only useful marginally while some are just flat out marketing gimmicks.

## *Conjugated Linoleic Acid*

CLA is one of those magic pills come true. Once consumed it burns off all fat and stimulates muscle growth. CLA is a fat that is mostly found in meat and dairy.

All of the above is 100% true....for rodents. That's right! CLA was initially tested on rodents and the results were hugely encouraging. Unfortunately, tests done on humans are completely inconclusive since, surprise, the human body is just a tad more complex than a rat's.

Those spammy ads you see promising a magic pill are usually CLA mixed with some other junk. Needless to say, you really don't need this.

## *Glutamine*

This one is a staple at any fitness store and online health store. Sadly, many trainers have drunk the kool-aid on this one. The reasoning for glutamine being necessary is sound enough.

Patients suffering heave burn injuries or muscle loss via disease are treated with doses of glutamine. This is an amino acid and patients experience remarkable recovery in their musculature. However, glutamine only seems to work when the level of muscle loss is excessive.

No matter how much of a beast you are in the gym, you simply will not suffer the level of muscle loss necessary to make glutamine useful.

## Garcinia Cambogia

This one is a popular "mystery herb" which promises extreme fat loss via a "weird" trick. The reality is you're just eating something that tastes funny and has an exotic name.

There have not been any studies showing the effectiveness of this so stay away from it.

## Green Coffee Bean Extract

Yet another magical fat burner. The reason this one deserves a place on this list, instead of the other one despite being a fat burner, is the eternal promise of the green coffee bean as if its something special.

As explained previously, fat burners are not meant to burn fat. They just give you a shot of energy and off you go to the gym. This works much the same way but the green coffee bean part is used to justify higher prices.

As mentioned in the previous section on fat burners, a cup of black coffee works just as well prior to a fasted workout.

Deer Antler Spray

You can't be serious...

Nitric Oxide

This is actually a well-meaning supplement but just not that effective or even necessary when it comes down to it.

Nitric Oxide is a necessary chemical which aids in our overall well being and health. Its just that if you follow a good diet, like the keto diet, and have your share of vegetables, you're probably getting all the nitric oxide you need.

So you really don't need this in pill form.

### *Calcium*

Yet another big one! Calcium is often marketed as being necessary for our bones and for the longest time, this was believed to be true. While it is correct that our bones are made of calcium, it does not follow that ingesting calcium in a pill form is going to aid bone strength.

In fact, many nutritionists and doctors have proposed that excessive calcium supplementation leads to calcification of our bones. In short, this is not something you want.

### *Specialized Protein*

You'll often see supplements like beef protein or chicken protein or some such. If you're vegan, it makes sense to purchase a vegan protein powder but even in this case, a pill doesn't make sense.

For the non-vegans, a regular whey or casein protein supplement does the job, you really don't need to worry about the superiority of beef protein versus turkey or chicken. If you really are fanatical about this, go eat a steak.

Stay away from the powders and pills.

This concludes our look at the world of supplements. As you can see, there are many options but the thing to remember above all else is that they are not strictly required (with a few exceptions) unless there are special conditions or goals you have. Above all else, this should guide your decision making.

# CHAPTER 5:

## EXERCISE AND WORKOUTS

Much like nutrition and our bodies' reaction to it, exercise and its role is something that is often filled with pseudoscience and hearsay. Just like diets, there are a number of options to choose from and it always seems like adopting one approach means sacrificing another. Most people end up losing perspective of the basic rule of exercise which is: just do something.

You need to do something every day that helps you break a sweat. This is the true role of exercise. Specialized workouts exist only for athletes who operate a very specialized level. For over 95% of people, a general workout which follows basic principles does the job. As we did in the nutrition chapters of this book, we're going to go back to basics and look at the different categories into which all exercises fall into.

It is important to state this at this point: There is no such thing as "the best fat burning exercise". This is because fat loss depends almost entirely on nutrition. As mentioned previously, you can lose weight without exercise but it's better not to. All exercise will help you burn fat, some better than others. What matters most is that you're doing something so don't worry too much about missing out on some special routine's benefits by doing something else.

## TYPES OF EXERCISE

Broadly speaking exercise can be classified into categories depending on the nature of the exercise or based on the goals you want to achieve with the exercise. Let's first look at classifying them on the basis of nature.

In this method, we can divide all forms of exercise into aerobic and anaerobic exercise. The difference between the two all comes down to oxygen as we shall see.

### *Aerobic Exercise*

In aerobic exercise, the heart pumps out oxygenated blood out to the muscles that are working. Put in a simpler way, running, cycling, swimming, dancing, hiking and the like when performed at a low intensity, that is, where you're going along at a decent pace but not sprinting, is aerobic exercise. When you hear people referring to cardio in the gym, this is what they mean. Aerobic exercise has a number of health benefits for both our breathing and cardiovascular systems as a whole.

You see, our heart is a muscle and its job is to pump oxygenated blood to all parts of our body. The lungs, when you inhale, provide this oxygen and as the oxygen is delivered to the heart, it pumps this out along with blood to our body in order for it to function. The stronger our heart is, the more it can pump on a single beat (which is simply the contraction and expansion process of the pump). This increased efficiency is a good thing as our heart needs to work less to produce greater results.

This is why, if you're unfit or don't exercise much, your resting heart rate will be higher than someone who exercises more. Your heart, if unfit, has to do a lot more work to perform at the same level as the person who exercises. This is also why at a lower level of physical exertion, compared to a person who is fitter, you run out of breath because your heart simply cannot keep up with your oxygen demands.

Aerobic exercise trains your lungs and your heart to pump oxygen more efficiently. As you exercise, your lungs are put to the test and their ability to take more air in and deliver the oxygen to the heart is tested. Once the oxygen is delivered, you are demanding a higher level of performance from your heart, via exercise, and the heart has to pump faster and more efficiently to meet your demands.

This oxygen once delivered to the muscles is used to burn fuel. As we saw previously, fuel is either glucose or fat and whichever is present is burned to fuel your muscles and produce performance. The thing about burning fat as fuel is that, being denser than glucose, it requires a greater amount of oxygen to burn. In turn, fat release a greater amount of energy, 9kcal per gram as opposed to 4 kcal per gram of glucose, as we saw in the very first chapter.

What all this means is that if you're on a keto diet and performing aerobic exercise, you're forcing your heart to pump more oxygen in order to burn fat. This trains your heart to be more efficient and it also ends up burning off your fat at a faster rate. As an aside, this is why what you eat matters more than how you exercise. Since all exercise produces the same effect on the heart, that is it needs to deliver oxygen to the muscles more efficiently, fat loss really comes down to this: is your body burning glucose or fat? The more fat it burns, the leaner you become. Hence, remove the glucose and force your body to burn the fat. The removal of glucose is entirely down to your diet.

Aerobic exercise also forces your muscles to consume the oxygen delivered to them more efficiently. The reason you get better at exercising the more you do it because your muscles have adapted to consuming oxygen and fuel more efficiently. This consumption is referred to as VO2. It is expressed in units of ml/kg per minute. Your body's VO2 max is the optimum rate at which your muscles can effectively utilize what is delivered to them. Keep this term in mind since we'll revisit it in the section on anaerobic exercise.

Aerobic exercise also has great psychological effects by helping reduce anxiety and depression. IN short, aerobic exercise simply makes you feel good!

So all of this sounds great so far and to be frank it is mostly so. There are some drawbacks to aerobic exercise from the perspective of someone who's looking at building all round health. Aerobic exercise is the best way to build your endurance, that is your body's ability to enhance its VO2. It is not a great way to build strength, that is, to increase the size of your muscles.

The more aerobic exercise you do, the more your body adapts. Your muscles adapt into the form best suited to consume oxygen as efficiently and as quickly as possible in order to fuel you for longer. This adaptation results in a base level of strength or a minimum required level of strength, beyond which the muscles prioritize burning fuel more efficiently. This is why, if you watch the Olympics, you will notice the physique of long-distance athletes is quite frail. Some of them, if they're reasonably tall, appear almost emaciated. Marathon runners tend to have a similar, slim physique. While such athletes have an incredible cardiovascular ability, being able to perform at high speed over incredibly long distances, they are not quite barometers of strength.

As an everyday Joe, you're probably more concerned with looking good than achieving God-like levels of cardio performance. Thus while it pays to engage in aerobic exercise, you need to supplement it with anaerobic exercise as well.

### Anaerobic Exercise

Anaerobic exercise, as the name suggests, refers to exercises performed where your body lacks oxygen or where your heart simply is able to deliver oxygen fast enough to your muscles. This sounds less like anaerobic and more like "inducing death" but this is actually a great way to train your heart and muscles.

Anaerobic exercises are performed at very high intensity since the aim is to deplete oxygen stores. Almost any aerobic activity can be made anaerobic by performing it faster. For example, if you were to cycle on a mountainous road at a pace more appropriate for the Tour de France, you're engaging in anaerobic exercise. Cycling in a park at a leisurely pace would be aerobic exercise.

So why is anaerobic exercise good for you? You see, as oxygen stores deplete, your muscles are forced to look elsewhere for fuel sources. This forces them to burn their existing energy stores, which is usually accessed only in emergencies, and thus conditions your muscles to go longer and become stronger since their primary fuel source is cut off.

As you can imagine, this state of things doesn't last very long. Anaerobic exercise is performed in short, sharp burst of activity, as opposed to aerobic exercise which is performed at low intensity for a longer period of time. Using the example of the Olympics, the 10,000-meter race is an aerobic activity whereas the 100-meter sprint is anaerobic.

Contrast the physiques of Olympic sprinters with the long distance runners and you'll see the sort of results anaerobic exercise produces. Aside from this, there are other benefits too including high-intensity exercise in your routine. Your muscles will become stronger with anaerobic routines since they are forced to support you and perform despite a lack of oxygen. This forces them to adapt and the result is you gain a higher level of strength. In addition to this, your bones also become stronger and there is the usual psychological benefit as well.

The biggest benefit though is to your VO2 max which increases. In other words, your body's cardiovascular system as a whole becomes more efficient. Your lungs deliver oxygen to your heart faster, your heart becomes more efficient at pumping out oxygenated blood and your muscles learn to use every single unit of oxygen to burn fuel more efficiently. Thus your endurance level rises.

It must be noted that though your endurance improves, it will not reach the levels it can if employing aerobic exercise. Think of it this way: Usain Bolt, being as great as he is, is not winning any medals in the 10,000-meter race. In fact, it'll be quite an achievement if he even qualifies for the finals. His body is optimized to deliver energy in short sharp bursts, not at a constant rate over long periods.

This higher intensity is also ideal for fat loss, compared to aerobic exercise. Due to the strain produced in your body while performing anaerobic exercises, your body remains in fuel burning mode for far longer than it would be performing aerobic exercise. If you're on the keto diet, this is excellent news since you'll burn even more fat given the glycogen depletion you induce via your diet.

There are obvious drawbacks to anaerobic exercise though. Aside from a lower level of endurance and the mentally taxing nature of it, if performed over a long session, it will result in muscle depletion. This is because once the energy stored within your muscles are depleted, your body has no choice but to burn your muscles for energy. Thus it is extremely easy to overtrain if you're not keenly aware of your session times.

Anaerobic exercise is not a great option for beginners since its demanding nature requires you to have a base level of strength and endurance for it to be effective. In the beginning, you probably won't be able to even approach the intensity levels required. Thus, it is best, as a beginner, to perform aerobic exercises first and then gradually build up to anaerobic ones.

So this is the way to categorize exercises based on their physiological functions. The other way we can classify exercise is via our goals, that is, do we wish to maximize strength or endurance? On the surface, this seems to be the same as aerobic versus anaerobic exercise but strength training has a key element we haven't looked at as yet and that is weight training.

Weight training is an extremely versatile method and can be geared towards both aerobic and anaerobic. This topic is, however, the one most plagued by pseudoscience and misinformation. Given the extreme lack of clarity, it is a good idea to dive into the basics of weight training and examining how it can help you achieve goals in both the strength and endurance department. We will also look at things like sets and rep ranges and what range produces what type of results. If you have no idea what a set or a rep is, don't worry, this will all be covered shortly.

## WEIGHT TRAINING BASICS

Weight training, as mentioned previously, is an extremely versatile way to increase your strength and endurance. It bears mentioning at this point that, the best way of increasing your endurance is via aerobic exercise or cardio. When training with weights you will find that most endurance exercises are of the anaerobic, high-intensity kind. Let's first see how weight training can improve your strength.

### *Strength Training*

If there's one workout philosophy that will benefit you the most, it is strength training. Simply put, as long as you eat right and train for strength, you will lose fat, build muscle and feel better. Even if you are female or vegan or whatever, this works for everyone. Simply put, the stronger you are, the easier everything is. Hopefully, that needs no explanation.

Secondly, one of the many benefits of strength training is the boost it gives your metabolism. The reason for this is that strength training affects something called EPOC or Excess Post-exercise Oxygen Consumption. This is the amount of oxygen your body needs to bring itself back to where it was prior to your workout. This recovery period can last for a while after your workout, depending on how strenuous it was, and while recovering your body continues to burn excess calories.

The more anaerobic your workout is, the greater the EPOC and the greater the number of calories you will burn post workout. Strength training is one of the best ways of achieving this due to the very nature of workouts. Here's what the American Council on Exercise has to say about this, via their website: **(MCCALL, 2019)**[1]

*Strength training with compound, multijoint weightlifting exercises or doing a weightlifting circuit that alternates between upper- and lower-body movements places a greater demand on the involved muscles for ATP from the anaerobic pathways. Increased need for anaerobic ATP*

---

[1] McCall, P. (2019). 7 Things to Know About Excess Post-exercise Oxygen Consumption (EPOC). Retrieved from https://www.acefitness.org/education-and-resources/professional/expert-articles/5008/7-things-to-know-about-excess-post-exercise-oxygen-consumption-epoc

*also creates a greater demand on the aerobic system to replenish that ATP during the rest intervals and the post-exercise recovery process. Heavy training loads or shorter recovery intervals increase the demand on the anaerobic energy pathways during exercise, which yields a greater EPOC effect during the post-exercise recovery period.*

The same article **(MCCALL, 2019)**[2] further points out:

*In an extensive review of the research literature on EPOC, Bersheim and Bahr (2003) concluded that "studies in which similar estimated energy cost or similar exercising VO2 have been used to equate continuous aerobic exercise and intermittent resistance exercise, have indicated that resistance exercise produces a greater EPOC response." For example, one study found that when aerobic cycling (40 minutes at 80 percent Max HR), circuit weight training (4 sets/8 exercises/15 reps at 50 percent 1-RM) and heavy resistance exercise (3 sets/8 exercises at 80-90 percent 1-RM to exhaustion) were compared, heavy resistance exercise produced the biggest EPOC.*

---

[2] McCall, P. (2019). 7 Things to Know About Excess Post-exercise Oxygen Consumption (EPOC). Retrieved from https://www.acefitness.org/education-and-resources/professional/expert-articles/5008/7-things-to-know-about-excess-post-exercise-oxygen-consumption-epoc

Strength training also has been shown to help manage and improve the quality of life for people with the following diseases:

## Osteoporosis

A study found that bone density increased even in elderly patients following a program of strength training **(VERACITY, 2019)**[3].

**FROM THE ARTICLE (VERACITY, 2019):**

*Numerous studies demonstrate strength training's ability to increase bone mass, especially spinal bone mass. According to Keeton, a research study by Ontario's McMaster University found that a year-long* **STRENGTH** *training program increased the spinal bone mass of postmenopausal women by nine percent. Furthermore, women who do not participate in strength training actually experience a decrease in* **BONE DENSITY**.

## Parkinson's Disease

A study conducted at the University of Illinois at Chicago concluded that strength training significantly improved the

---

[3] Veracity, D. (2019). Bone density sharply enhanced by weight training, even in the elderly. Retrieved from
https://www.naturalnews.com/010528_bone_density_mineral.html

motor skills of patients with Parkinson's disease(**"LONG-TERM WEIGHT TRAINING MAY BENEFIT PARKINSON'S DISEASE PATIENTS", 2019)** [4]

## *Lymphedema*

A study carried out on breast cancer survivors concluded that strength training resulted in *"a decreased incidence of exacerbations of lymphedema, reduced symptoms, and increased strength"* (**SCHMITZ ET AL., 2009)**[5].

FIBROMYALGIA: (**HÄKKINEN A ET AL., 2001)**[6].

CANCER SURVIVORS: (**DE BACKER ET AL., 2007)**[7].

---

[4] Long-term weight training may benefit Parkinson's disease patients. (2019). Retrieved from https://www.news-medical.net/news/20120217/Long-term-weight-training-may-benefit-Parkinsons-disease-patients.aspx

[5] Schmitz, K., Ahmed, R., Troxel, A., Cheville, A., Smith, R., & Lewis-Grant, L. et al. (2009). Weight Lifting in Women with Breast-Cancer–Related Lymphedema. *New England Journal Of Medicine, 361*(7), 664-673. doi: 10.1056/nejmoa0810118

[6] Häkkinen A, Häkkinen K, Hannonen P, et al. Strength training induced adaptations in neuromuscular function of premenopausal women with fibromyalgia: comparison with healthy women. *Annals of the Rheumatic Diseases* 2001;60:21-26.

[7] De Backer, I., Van Breda, E., Vreugdenhil, A., Nijziel, M., Kester, A., &

As should be evident by now, strength training's benefits go beyond mere physical changes.

## *Workouts*

Strength training workouts tend to be of higher intensity, but this doesn't mean you're running around all the time. It just means you'll be lifting close to your maximum effort every time you lift a weight. Getting started in strength training is easy. You simply do all the exercises listed below for the indicated sets and reps.

A rep stands for repetitions and is the number of times you will be lifting the weight. A set is simply one set of how many ever reps you choose to do together prior to resting. Strength training workouts usually have 5 sets of 5 reps for each exercise or 3X5 (3 sets of 5 reps).

So if you're going to squat 5X5, this means you squat 5 times then rest, then 5 times again and rest and repeat this three more times. In 3X5, you'll be squatting for 5 reps three separate times.

---

Schep, G. (2007). High-intensity strength training improves quality of life in cancer survivors. *Acta Oncologica, 46*(8), 1143-1151. doi: 10.1080/02841860701418838

As for the list of exercises you need to do, there is a very small number. While the correct form for these exercises is beyond the scope of this book, you can find excellent videos and articles on how to execute them correctly. It is best to begin with an empty barbell and master your form before progressing further. The exercises you will need to do are:

- Squats (back or front)

- Overhead Barbell Press

- Deadlift

- Bench Press

- Barbell Rows

That's it! You will not be doing all of these exercises at once in the same workout session. Instead, you will just perform the squat and rotate the other exercises around it for 3 days or 4 days per week.

There are many resources available online for you to design a strength training workout revolving around these five exercises. One of the benefits of strength training is that the workout is very simple to design and follow since there aren't many movements you're doing. They are also brutally effective since all these movements are total body workouts and thus burn the most calories which in turn means greater fat loss as your performance on them increases.

You might have heard of people complaining about injuries via strength and weight training. This is because all these exercises are technical in nature and you should always perform them with proper form. Getting injured by practicing poor form and blaming the exercise for being dangerous is a lot like driving down the wrong side of the road and blaming your car for the ensuing accident.

Women have special blocks to strength training, or training like a man, as many seem to think. Here's the deal: if you train like a man, you'll look like a goddess. There's no workout in this world that can make you look like a man unless you take an ungodly amount of steroids. Eat right and train hard and you'll look leaner and be stronger. Being strong does not mean having bulging muscles like a bodybuilder! Neither does it mean you'll look like the women in bodybuilding magazines. As mentioned earlier, looking like that requires you to ingest steroids and nothing in here calls for that.

## *Training for Shape*

Weights can be used to tone your muscles and give them a desirable shape as well. While strength training focuses on building raw strength, there isn't much it does in the way of aesthetics beyond making you look leaner. In other words, you will not be able to have an 8 pack of abs via strength training alone. You will look fit but lack the definition you often see in images of celebrities and fitness models.

Some people are perfectly happy with this of course and there is no rule that says you need to look like a fitness model. There are some though who prefer to have a lot of definition in their muscles. Once you've built up your strength to an intermediate level, you can then begin to focus on toning your muscles and achieving a pleasing aesthetic look.

To do this you will have to perform what is called isolation exercises. While strength training focuses on total body movements, isolation movements are focused on just one portion of muscles, like the chest, shoulder, calves and so on.

Exercises for strength are done free, with just weight balanced on a barbell. Isolation exercises usually involve dumbells and machines. The number of sets is lower than on strength training exercises but the number of reps is higher, usually in the 8-12 range. So you will be performing sets of 3X12 or 2X15 even (3 sets of 12 reps and 2 sets of 15 reps).

Once you reach an appropriate level, you can cycle between strength training and higher rep training to ensure gains in both areas. The exercises that you can do under this sort of training are numerous, too numerous in fact to list out here, but even a simple search online will yield favorable results.

As for rotating, ideally, you want to perform one or two strength training exercises and then supplement them with the higher rep exercises. This will cause an increase in the number of days you have to go to the gym since you'll have to extend your strength training out to an extra day. However, combined with a cardio session at the end this is an excellent fat burning workout.

## *Cardio and Endurance Training*

Cardiovascular training or simply cardio is relatively straight forward. There are two types of cardio, broadly speaking, steady state and high intensity. Steady state cardio is essentially aerobic exercise while HIIT is anaerobic. Again, aerobic and anaerobic exercise doesn't just involve cardio.

While starting out it is best to perform steady state cardio after your strength workouts. You don't need to overdo it, a period of 10-15 minutes is more than enough. Once your workouts rise in intensity, you'll find 10 minutes more than adequate.

You can choose to jog, cycle, swim or hop on the elliptical machine in your gym. Make sure to get your heart rate up to around to 50% of your maximum heart rate. You can calculate this by subtracting your age from 220. 50% of that resulting number is what you want to aim at in your cardio sessions.

Once you've built up a base standard of strength and endurance you can start experimenting with interval training or HIIT. HIIT stands for High-Intensity Interval Training and is an anaerobic form of exercise. HIIT combined with strength training will give you the maximum amount of fat loss possible.

It is, however, extremely taxing mentally when you first begin. The structure of a HIIT workout goes something like this. You exercise at full speed for an interval and then rest for an interval. You repeat this sequence over a period of 10-15 minutes. If you're doing HIIT at the end of your workout, its best to stick to just 10 minutes or else you'll risk muscle loss and excessive stress buildup.

The work and rest interval lengths are usually in a ratio of 1:2 when you begin. So if you work for one minute you rest for two. You need to really crank up your activity level and get your heart rate at least 80% of your maximum heart rate. This will be difficult to do at first so it's better to choose intervals of a minute which will allow you to build up to that level. Your aim should be to get there as fast as possible, not get there at the 58th second.

Once you have a measure of how soon you can get your heart rate up, you adjust your work interval length and rest interval accordingly and as you progress you shorten the rest interval until the ratio is inverted. That is, you'll be working twice as long as you rest. Another advanced option is to opt for Tabata intervals. Beginners to HIIT are cautioned against adopting this because of the issue of getting your heart rate up. Tabata intervals tend to be short and most beginners aren't used to the extreme activity levels HIIT demands.

Handling the mental stress is perhaps the toughest part of HIIT. The levels of exhaustion you will experience is unlike anything else due to the extreme demands being placed on you. As a rule of thumb, if you aren't completely exhausted, you're probably not pushing hard enough. As you can imagine, doing all this fasted (on CKD) is extremely taxing.

If you choose to do just HIIT, an optimal workout time limit is 20 minutes. You can choose just about any activity to perform be it cycling, sprinting or even hopping on the elliptical machine. Swimming is not recommended for obvious reasons unless it's a shallow pool or you're an extremely good swimmer. You can perform HIIT using weights as well. A back squat or front squat with low weights will do the job but this is advisable only if you're extremely confident and proficient with your mechanics. The last thing you want to do is injure yourself.

## *The Ideal Workout*

You might as well know this right off the bat: the ideal workout doesn't exist. The best workout to perform is one that challenges you to push your limits and more often than not leaves you energized at the end of it. There will be times when you will be exhausted but overall, if your workouts are pumping you up and improving your quality of life, then you're doing things correctly.

Most people expect instant results and when they don't see the changes in the mirror they get upset and lose motivation. As mentioned earlier it will take at least three months for physical changes to show up. Resist the temptation to chop and change due to thinking the grass is greener on the other side. Pick a workout routine that feels good and stick to it.

The more you keep things simple, the easier it will be for you to follow your routines. A lot of beginners tend to sabotage themselves by adopting new routines and adding and removing things all the time in the hope of getting better results. The reality is that fat loss and good fitness is simple and has been complicated thanks to erroneous knowledge and marketing.

Your body is not a snowflake so go ahead and test it rigorously. You'll be pleasantly surprised by the results you achieve.

## *Other Workouts*

It isn't necessary for you to take up weight training of course. If you feel more comfortable running or swimming then feel free to do so. Just remember that adding muscle will help increase your performance in those activities too. At the very least, two days aimed at muscle building per week is a good idea. This way you get to do what you like and you're helping hasten your fat loss as well.

There are a lot of new training methods out there like Zumba these days which make for fun workouts. While these are great to partake in, remember that they don't build muscle beyond a certain point and if you stick only to them, you will hit a fat loss plateau and won't break past it because your body just doesn't have enough muscle to justify burning more fat.

The more muscle you have, the lesser the need for body fat so it is essential you focus on this as mentioned previously, at a minimum for 2 days per week.

Now that we've looked at training, let's combine this knowledge with what we know about the keto diet and see how you can marry the two together.

# CHAPTER 6:

## TRAINING PLANS

The type of training you choose to do will be dictated by the diet plan you choose to follow. If you're a beginner, for example, the SKD will fit you the best and as far as training goes, it's best to start off with something you're familiar with and comfortable doing. However, you will eventually have to shift your training to a slightly higher gear to continue to make progress and lose fat.

This chapter is going to give you a full training plan based on the diet you choose to follow and also how this will affect your performance and goals.

## SKD TRAINING PLANS

On the SKD you'll be following a pretty straightforward nutrition scheme. As long as you keep your carbs low and fat high, you'll be in ketosis and make progress. Given the abrupt switch though it's probably a good idea to take things slow and ease into training, even if you're someone who's used to training a lot. Let's break it down on a weekly basis and look at what you can expect and how you can tailor your training accordingly.

## Week 1

Week 1 begins with you adopting the keto diet. Ideally, you should do this over a weekend or two consecutive non-training days. You should have your macros figured out in advance and have everything ready to go. We'll go over your meal plan later so don't fret if you're worried about planning your meals.

The first week is usually characterized by the dreaded keto fog. You will feel lethargic and sluggish and you won't be able to sleep very well. The first week is also where you will lose a lot of weight. However, this is just excess water being drained since you're restricting carbs.

In light of this, you should ensure your water intake is high since you will be shedding a lot of it and your body hasn't fully adjusted to using less water than is usually available. Also, it's a good idea to go slow in training this week. You should be keenly aware of getting exhausted and overtraining and not exceed these limits.

Don't be discouraged by the drop-in training performance, you'll make it back within a week's time. While you need to be aware of lethargy and a general lack of energy, resist the temptation to skip training altogether. Training forces your body even more to burn fat instead of glucose and will bring you into ketosis faster. The faster you enter ketosis, the quicker you'll be rid of the mental fog.

This doesn't mean you train like a maniac. Go easy and find a good balance. This is also the first time you'll be maintaining a caloric deficit. The keto diet takes some adjusting to mentally at first because you'll be eating a far lesser quantity of food than you're accustomed to, even if you're eating the same number of calories. Remember, a gram of fat releases 9kcal of energy as opposed to 4 kcal per gram for carbs.

Therefore, it's logical that you'll need to eat lesser fat to gain the same amount of energy as carbs. Your meal sizes will shrink and you'll probably second guess yourself because of this. Always monitor your mood. If you're feeling lethargic, this is normal. If you feel short tempered and stressed out and find yourself irritated constantly, you've made a mistake calculating your macros and need to eat more food.

For those of you who will be training for the first time, pick an activity you've always wanted to do and start doing it. Running, swimming, playing a sport, cycling, whatever it is, just start moving and breaking a sweat. If you'll be hitting the gym, stick to the treadmills, ellipticals and stationary bikes for now and perform these exercises for 45 minutes at a comfortable speed. The key is to ease yourself into this new regime and not shock yourself into it.

You will feel sore after your workout and this is good. This is how your body becomes stronger and fitter. During the first week, it's best if you train on alternate days for 3 or 4 days. Pick any time of the day that is convenient for you and always eat a meal within an hour of finishing training.

## *Week 2*

You should be back to normal by this time or towards the end of the previous week. If you're still having problems, try working out fasted for a day to see if your body adjusts. If you're still having issues there are two possible issues. Either you've miscalculated your macros and are eating far too less or your body is simply refusing to adjust due to some condition you are not aware of. If it's the latter case, consult your doctor immediately and act as they advise.

If you're back to normal levels, this is great news! You can continue training the way you have been, prior to adopting the diet. If you were not training before, continue what you were doing on week 1. If you feel up to it, try increasing the length of your workout or increase the number of days while keeping the same workout length.

This week is all about feeling good and observing how you're adapting to your new diet. So keep working near your limit while simultaneously discovering how much you can push against it.

As a reminder, you'll be performing aerobic cardio activities this week as well. It's still too soon to transition to weight training.

## Week 3

This is the week where you will first begin to push your limits and really start testing yourself. This doesn't have to be strenuous, mind you. If you find yourself becoming irritable or stressed out, remember, this means you're eating too less and have miscalculated your macros. So always be on the lookout for this.

By this point, you will have noticed that you feel hungry most of the time. This is not a rabid hunger but your stomach will feel lighter than usual and your brain will keep telling you that you can accommodate a little more food in there. This is happening because you're in a caloric deficit. If you've never experienced this before, it will be a weird sensation for you to not eat when you're hungry.

Again, this is worth repeating: monitor your mood constantly. If you constantly feel stressed out and irritable or burned out, you're eating too less. If this is the case eat more. Your hunger should not be more than a mild one. If you had to put words to it it would probably be "I could eat more but I can manage this".

From a training perspective, this week is when you will need to start lifting weights. Ideally, you will begin a strength training program of your choice. When picking a program, remember the guidelines set out in the previous chapter and pick something that is simple and easy to follow and incorporates progressive overload principles. You will be starting light, with an empty bar, so take it easy and continue as you previously were with your aerobic exercise.

Also, limit your workouts to 4 days per week. Recovery is where the most progress is made NOT during workouts. Most beginners fail to recognize this and workout to insane schedules. Rest and recovery are as essential as working out. Rest when you're supposed to and workout when you should. Discipline is not just performing an action when you need to but also involves doing nothing when the time is called for it.

## Week 4

You're well into ketosis by now and you should be seeing its effect on the weighing scale. If you aren't seeing any progress, don't worry. You're probably not maintaining enough of a deficit. So reduce your meal portions a bit and see how that works. On the other hand, if you find you've gained weight, you're obviously eating too much to reduce your portions and monitor how that goes.

As far as workouts go, you should be well established into a schedule by now. Your strength training will be to approach challenging levels by the end of this week and you will begin to feel exhausted by your workouts. This is a good time to reduce your aerobic exercises and limit them to perhaps 10-15 minutes at the most after your workout.

You might be bummed out by this if you really love cycling or running but this will pay dividends in the long run so stick to the method. Your increased strength will give you more energy to perform better at those activities.

## Week 5

This is where your training becomes very challenging and most people will start stalling on their weights at this point. This represents literally the first time your body has hit its limits and is now pushing past them so its a time to celebrate!

You should have a handle on your diet by now in terms of eyeballing how much you need to eat to maintain your macros and you should have a rough idea of whether you've eaten the correct amount by observing your hunger pangs, the degree of them that is.

If you feel up to it, try alternating between HIIT and steady state cardio at the end of your workouts. If HIIT is too strenuous, leave it be. Remember, your HIIT workout should last a maximum of 10 minutes.

## *Week 6*

By this point, you should have lost at least 4 pounds of fat and your body weight should reflect this. If you're examining yourself in the mirror, you should see changes in the areas where you usually don't accumulate fat. These areas are usually the ones which tone up first.

Given the strength training you're doing, you should be seeing some physical changes from that as well. If you're squatting correctly, you will notice your legs becoming thicker and stronger. Your upper back will also have some definition by now and the deadlifts will have affected your posterior quite a bit by now.

At this point, it is crucial to continue observing your body and most importantly, identify the differences between being sore and an injury. Sometimes, in the excitement of all these changes, you will push a little too hard and tweak something. When you're sore, you will find it hard to move the muscle and there will be some pain but if you perform the movement that produced the soreness, you'll find that it goes away.

With an injury, the pain is constant and performing the movement only makes it worse. Those of you performing the bench press for the first time will feel this soreness in your chest. Don't mistake this for an injury. If you continue to perform the movement, it'll go away.

## Week 7

By this point, you should have lost at least 5 pounds if you've done things correctly. If not, tweak your macros and observe what is helping and what is hindering and act accordingly.

If you've been experimenting with HIIT, you should be finding it a bit easier by now. Continue to push the limits by testing the work and rest interval timings. If you find HIIT a challenge but not an overwhelming one, you can drop steady state cardio at this point. This has the added benefit of reducing your overall workout time as well.

## Week 9

Yes, we've skipped a week since by this point things should be in control for you. Hopefully, you've reached a stage where you're stalling for a second time in your strength training.

This is also the point where you will observe that you're losing lesser weight at a slower rate than previously. This is a very good sign if it happens because it means you've reached a stage where the most stubborn fat is clinging onto you. Once this fat leaves, there's not much more left!

The reason this happens is that you've lost enough weight to throw off your macros and your deficit. You see, since you're at a lower weight, your BMR is at a lower level and your deficit is lower. So simply recalculate your ratios and off you go!

This is how you handle the dreaded fat loss plateau which you may have read about. Most people make the mistake of increasing their activity level but remember what we learned earlier. Fat loss is almost entirely dependent on your diet, not your workout routine.

What has also happened is that your body has become much more efficient at producing fuel for itself, so it is using whatever food you provide a lot more efficiently. The more efficient it becomes, the more it does with less. This does not mean you can indiscriminately reduce your food intake, of course.

### *Week 10*

This is the point where all those around you will start noticing changes in you since they've become obvious by now. You'll need to start replacing your wardrobe soon!

Jokes apart, you simply need to stay the course at this point and just keep doing what you're doing.

## *Week 12*

We're nearing the 3-month mark now and its time to take stock of your situation. You've probably lost around 10 pounds of fat by now. You're maintaining a healthy caloric deficit with your diet. You should be around the intermediate level with your strength training.

At this point, with regards to strength training, a beginner level routine will not help you much and you face a choice to either start an intermediate routine or maintain your levels and instead add other activities you enjoy. So if you've had to give up some cycling or swimming to train in the gym more, this is the time you pick that back up.

You reduce your strength training in the gym to 3 days and lift the same weight as close to your stalling points as possible and indulge in the other activities. You will find a marked improvement in those given the changes you've made.

Alternatively, you can continue on an intermediate program and add some split training routines. If you do this you will have to increase the number of days you train. Also, remember to keep doing your HIIT or steady state cardio, whichever it is you find useful.

Given that your body has been on a deficit for three months, its time to allow it to recover a bit. You see, being on a deficit for longer than this not healthy. So recalculate your macros and start eating at maintenance levels and always keep a track of your body weight. If you find yourself putting on weight, you're eating too much. If you're losing weight, you're eating too less. Your weight should stay the same more or less within a pound. You need to eat at maintenance for a couple of months and then get back onto a deficit to further cut fat if you need to.

Alternatively, if you're happy with the way you look, you can try bulking up via the HPKD or TKD and increase your muscle mass.

Either way, congratulations! You've discovered how simple weight loss and fat loss really is!

# CHAPTER 7:

## HPKD TRAINING PLAN

We've looked at the aims of the HPKD previously and how, if your objective is to increase the amount of muscle, that is to bulk up, the HPKD is the best diet for you to follow. With this diet you will be running a caloric surplus, that is you will be eating more than your maintenance level requires.

This caloric excess does not mean you have a free license to eat any old junk. You still need to follow the basic of good nutrition and watch what you eat. The HPKD is more fun to follow than the SKD though due to this reason.

We'll now take a look at your training plan on a weekly basis. There are some assumptions which have been made here. One is that if you're looking to bulk up, you've already had some experience training and know your way around a gym. While your experience doesn't have to be extensive, you can start strength training immediately and don't need to perform aerobic cardio to increase your base strength.

If this is not the case, the SKD is recommended for you since you probably don't have the muscle to begin with and will probably end up with middling results by following this diet routine.

So having made that clear, let's dive in!

## HPKD TRAINING PLANS

Since the HPKD calls for maintaining an excess of calories, you won't find this very taxing mentally. However, you will need to hit the gym hard and regularly because those excess calories, if not burned to fuel muscles, will turn into fat, defeating the purpose of following the diet in the first place.

### *Week 1*

Just like with the SKD, the best way to begin the HPKD is by adopting it over a weekend or over two non-training days to give yourself ample time to adjust to the new diet regime. Prior to beginning its best to have all your supplements sorted out, especially fiber supplements since the combination of higher protein and low carbs pretty much remove all fiber from your diet.

Your workouts should not be fasted under any circumstances. Since the aim of this diet is to aid in muscle gain, working out fasted will inhibit muscle growth. While there's no set time for you to workout, aim to do so on a full stomach.

Your workout themselves should be a combination of strength training, depending on your strength level this can be beginner or intermediate level programs, and isolation exercises. A word of caution though: if you're not yet at an intermediate level of strength then sticking to beginner strength program and building your strength up to intermediate standards is the best way forward.

Timing your cardio sessions is of great importance if you're looking to build muscle. To this effect, it's best to perform cardio prior to your workouts for around 10-15 minutes. Doing so after your workouts will only cause greater stress to be placed on your muscles and you will risk muscle loss, even if you're running a caloric surplus.

The only program to absolutely avoid is HIIT. You will be training at a pretty high-intensity level to begin with so HIIT would just be overkill and your gains will just take longer to be realized.

### Week 2

You should be fully adjusted to your new diet by now. If the keto fog still persists, take the same steps as advised while doing the SKD, that is, figure out if you've calculated your macros correctly and if so, then consult your doctor about the efficacy of the diet.

If you are properly adjusted then as far as your workout goes, its best to continue your current program and to keep progressively increasing the weight. Remember to finish your cardio pre-workout and do not do so post workout since this will limit your gains.

## Week 4

This is an important week in terms of taking stock of where your progress is at in terms of target weight and workout performance. This week marks a month since you started the diet and the first thing to measure is your weight.

Remember that by maintaining a caloric excess, you're targeting a gain of 1 pound per week. Now not all of this will be muscle but by eating healthy and closely following workout principles, you will minimize fat gain and maximize your muscle gains. So the first thing to see is whether you've been putting on weight as per expected guidelines.

If you find yourself below your projected weight at this point, you ought to increase the calories you're eating by around 250 kcal. If you're overweight, reduce your consumption by 250 kcal. Next, you need to determine whether this increased weight is fat or muscle predominantly.

You could do a body composition test which a lot of clinics offer and get it done scientifically. If this seems like overkill to you, an easy way to determine this is to look at your workouts. Are you lifting heavier weight than when you began? How much heavier? Have you stalled recently? Ideally, you wouldn't have stalled up until now and your lifting weight at a far higher level than when you began.

This is, perhaps, a more artistic method of determining fat vs muscle so don't be alarmed or overreact to whatever you find. It's still too early to determine all this and this is merely a checkpoint to make sure you're on track.

We'll cover more on the topic of tracking and measurement in a later chapter so you will understand how to measure and more importantly what and when to measure.

## Week 6

This week is when you'll begin stalling on your lifts and you will begin to find cardio a lot tougher to perform. If you find your stress levels increasing too much, to the extent that you're dreading your workouts, reduce your cardio sessions to once or twice a week.

Performing strength exercises at high intensity will build your anaerobic capacity so your cardio system will get a good workout. The idea is to maximize muscle gains which in turn will burn food more efficiently and reduce your fat gains. So always keep this objective in mind.

As for your lifts, a good idea to stimulate growth is to perform a single, heavy rep at the end of your sets. So if you're squatting 5X5, add a 6th set of 1 rep at the end with a weight that you think is too heavy, within a reasonable distance of where you're actually lifting right now. For example, if you're squatting 250 pounds and are close to stalling out, load 275 pounds on the bar. It's not necessary for you to actually squat this weight (if you think you can with the help of a spotter, do so) but at the very least balance it for a few seconds.

What this does is it gets your body and mind used to the idea that it can carry this much weight. A lot of weight lifting is mental and you'll be surprised at how much smoother your gains become by incorporating this technique.

Your diet should be on autopilot by now and you should be at the point where you can eyeball your portions and estimate whether it's too much or too less. It is essential for you to get adequate sleep and rest. Remember, muscle is gained, and fat is burned when you rest, not when you workout.

## Week 10

You will be approaching your second level of stalling on weights by this point. If you're not there yet, don't worry, you'll soon arrive. Once you stall and reload towards the weight again (every strength training program will explain what this is and how to do it. This is a diet book and hence, this process is beyond our scope), you will need to start planning our how you wish to take your training forward.

You could adopt an intermediate training program or, like in the SKD, you could maintain the weight levels and start engaging in other activities like cycling, running, sports etc. Either way, make sure you recalculate your macro levels and make sure you eat at maintenance.

You'll find your levels have changed and you will also need to factor in a higher activity level so do keep that in mind. Performing a full body composition test is a good idea at this point to determine how many pounds of muscle versus fat you have gained.

It bears mentioning at this point that those of you who have bulked on a carb-heavy diet will find that amount of muscle you have gained will be lesser than what you've observed previously. So why adopt the HPKD to bulk you might ask? This is a good question and it ultimately comes down to how well you think you can shed the fat you've gained during bulking.

If you find shedding the fat easy, then perhaps a carb heavy diet will be better suited for your bulk. However, if you have always struggled to shed the extra fat and during cutting, have always ended up losing muscle and ending up with a skinny fat look, then the HPKD will give you better results during the bulk since you'll be far more used to eating fat (as opposed to excess carbs) and your body will be completely adjusted to burning fat for fuel instead of having to re-adjust again.

If you're already at an advanced level and want to achieve the double advantage of losing fat and building muscle at the same time, then you need to get on the CKD or TKD. The CKD can be adopted by beginners as well who are having trouble getting adjusted to the high-fat requirements of the keto diet. We'll look at this next.

# CHAPTER 8:

## CKD AND TKD TRAINING PLANS

As we've seen previously, the CKD and TKD involve fueling yourself with carbs with an aim to replenish your glycogen stores to fuel your workouts or in the case o the CKD, to gently immerse yourself into the keto diet with an aim of going fully onto the SKD within a period of time.

Both objectives have very different goals and indeed, a very different audience. With this view, we will be looking at training plans for beginners, new to the keto diet, on the CKD and the training for more experienced people who can use either the CKD or TKD.

We'll first look at the beginners on the CKD

## BEGINNERS' CKD TRAINING PLAN

If you're new to the keto diet and are having troubles for whatever reason in adapting to the lesser carbs required or if you feel a gentler introduction to the keto diet would serve you better, then following the CKD for a period of 2-3 weeks is ideal.

As a refresher, the CKD calls for you to load on carbs on 2 days out of 7 and follow the SKD on the remaining 5. Since you're a beginner, you'll be maintaining a caloric deficit, no matter what you're eating so do keep that in mind.

### *Week 1*

You will need to calculate two sets of macros for the CKD, one for the carbs heavy days and one for the SKD days. Remember, carb loading doesn't mean you get to binge on whatever you want. The CKD plan doesn't allow you to have any cheat days so you will be maintaining a deficit on all 7 days (We'll talk about cheat days more in the next few chapters).

Ideally, you should have your carb days coincide with your final workout day for the week and the day right after that. Another good option is to have the first carb day coincide with the rest day prior to the final workout of the week and the 2nd carb day be the day of the final workout itself. This way, you're properly fueled for the workout and can begin to prepare to enter ketosis soon after.

Given the 2 days you'll be eating carbs, you should not have much of a keto fog effect going on. If you do still experience it, consult your doctor. Remember to monitor your stress and mood levels and see if you've calculated your macros correctly and are eating right.

For your workouts, if you've never exercised before, begin with steady state aerobic cardio activities for this week and the next. If you are more experienced than a rank beginner, you may begin strength training with an empty bar and start working your way up.

### Week 2

The second week of the CKD is pretty much the same as the previous one. You will continue to follow the diet guidelines and keep monitoring your mood and stress levels in case you're eating less.

If you were only performing cardio the previous week, continue to do so this week as well. You can try to increase the length of your workout for up to an hour this week. Don't worry if you can't go that long, the aim is to progressively increase your work levels.

You will be working out at least 4 days a week this week if you're not strength training.

## Week 3

This will be your final week eating carbs before switching fully over to the SKD. If you feel comfortable doing so earlier than this feel free to do so. This week the only major change you will be making is, you will be eating carbs only one day of the week. This will be the day of your final workout of the week.

Again, this is not an excuse to binge or think that this is a final meal of sorts and lose self-control. Monitor yourself the days after this carb meal and see how you're taking it and adjusting to the SKD full time.

If you're finding some levels of fog occurring, this is normal and will probably persist for a week, albeit its occurrence is pretty rare. If this fog lasts for a longer time than that, the keto diet is probably not for you and you should consult a doctor to get your symptoms checked out.

For those who are able to adjust successfully, which is usually the majority of people, you can start following the SKD from week 3 onwards in the previous chapter and also keep increasing your workout activities as per the guidelines explained in that chapter.

# TKD/CKD TRAINING PLAN

For more experienced people, that is those who are used to working out and have dieted in one form or another in the past, the TKD is a great option as opposed to an SKD due to the dual benefit of cutting fat and building muscle.

While you can adopt the CKD as well, your rate of fat loss will be low with this. The only exception is if you're a very experienced trainer, in which case you will hardly need a book to tell you what to do.

In the below sections, we'll address both options, the CKD and TKD, equally so you can get a better idea of which option might work for you best. Also, to make it abundantly clear, you will be eating at maintenance on this regime.

### *Week 1*

If you choose to follow the TKD, this week will be more challenging than on the CKD. Remember to consume only up to 30 g carbs prior to your workout and not more. The idea is to have the carbs fuel your workout and then post workout, have your body hasten back into ketosis as soon as possible.

The type of workout you choose to follow will dictate the amount of carbs you choose to consume pre-workout. A good idea is to track the number of calories you regularly burn as part of a typical workout and aim to eat enough carbs to cover 3/4ths of that.

If you're on the CKD, remember to consume lesser carbs on the second day than the first in order to push yourself into ketosis sooner. Generally, the CKD is a less efficient way of achieving the dual goal of increased muscle and lower fat so it is advisable to switch to the TKD is convenient. You will still hit your goals if done properly but it will just take longer.

## Week 3

Week 3 is a good point at which you can begin HIIT. As a rule, perform your cardio whenever you feel comfortable doing so and whichever gives you the best performance. Since you're in maintenance, it is not advisable to skip cardio since you might end up gaining some fat. As a rule of thumb, do steady state cardio prior to your workout and HIIT after your workout.

For those on CKD, you will need to be performing HIIT fasted the day after your second carb day. You can choose to do this in the morning and workout in the evening or combine the two into one morning workout. No approach is superior to another, so go with whatever works best for you.

This is also the point where, should you choose, you can switch over to the TKD. A pertinent question to consider here is are you better off working out fasted or not? The answer, again, is do whatever you can sustain for the longest. A fasted workout is mentally more taxing and while you can will your way through a few days or even weeks, eventually, it catches up to you. Consistency is what brings results so do whatever you can maintain the longest for.

## Week 6

You have probably stalled a couple times on your lifts by now and must be approaching your strength limits. Generally, it is not advisable at this point to change your activities. Instead, adopt an intermediate level strength program and follow that for more gains.

This applies to both CKD and TKD options. As always keep tracking your weight and if you're seeing any significant weight gain or loss, adjust your macros accordingly.

## Week 8

At this point, you should be seeing physical changes in the mirror. Keep doing what you're doing. To be perfectly honest, at an intermediate level, you will not see huge changes like those at a beginner's stage. It will be boring and that's perfectly OK.

## Week 12

At this point, you need to take stock of your gains and your goals. If need be, this is where you can choose to maintain your strength level and branch out into different activities like sports or cycling, running and other activities you usually enjoy. As always make sure to take your activity level into consideration when calculating your energy needs.

This concludes our look at the training plan and schedules with respect to the SKD, HPKD, TKD, and CKD. As you may have noticed, there are lesser things to worry about as you make progress largely because a lot of it becomes second nature to you. This is why persistence pays off and making progress will become second nature to you.

You will have noticed there are a quite a few things to track and this might be intimidating for you if you're just starting out. With this in mind, in the next chapter, we will take a look at everything to do with tracking and recording progress.

# CHAPTER 9:

## TRACKING

You will not make progress in anything that you do not track. When starting out, tracking will feel tedious because you've probably never bothered to do so. This chapter will give you everything you need to know about not just what to track, but also how and when to track them.

Without further ado, let's jump right in and look at the things you need to track from a diet perspective.

## DIET TRACKING

There are a few things you have to track when following your chosen keto diet. Some of them are obvious and some are not. The good news is from a diet perspective there really isn't all that much to do and most of it becomes repetitive after a couple weeks.

In fact, you'll probably be able to eyeball all of these without the need for any measuring because you'll get adjusted to it.

## Ingredient Portions

This is the major thing you need to track as part of any diet, not just keto. Your best investment with this view will be a food weighing scale. This way you will be able to measure your portions in grams or pounds.

Another good idea is to purchase measuring cups for fluids. Given the demands of the diet, you will be eating more cream and fatty oils so measuring these out is essential. Remember, you get a lot more energy from a gram of fat than carbs and protein so at first, you will not be able to eyeball how much you think you need.

## Calorie Count

Using any free calorie tracker (like FitDay for example) is absolutely necessary. Not only do these software make it easy for you to track your calories but they also help enforce discipline by forcing you to engage in your progress.

This really should be a no-brainer but you'd be surprised at the number of people who neglect this and squander all progress. Another rookie mistake that people make is to think that they need to enter food into this software every single day.

The key to making any diet regime work is to make it as repeatable and simple as possible. This means if you're comfortable with entering your food into this every time you eat, then great. If you find this tedious and irritating, then you need to set up your process to be as repeatable as possible. We'll look at this in greater detail in the next chapter but one way of doing this is to reduce the number of raw ingredients from which you will cook your meals to a small number.

This way you know the calorie counts of all the ingredients and cooking your meals simply becomes a case of mixing and matching them. Alternatively, you could simply eat the same thing every day for a while and when you get bored of it, change it up with a new set of ingredients and calculate your macros for the new foods.

### Mental State

While this is a bit nebulous to track, in that there are no numbers involved, it is just as important to track. Your levels of stress and moods are key indicators in helping you figure out whether you're headed in the right direction or not. If your caloric deficit is too high, this will always manifest as irritability and stress or the feeling of being burned out.

## *Ketone Levels*

Tracking your ketone levels is also a good idea since this will let you know how your body reacts specifically to certain types of food. Everyone is built differently and determining the number of carbs that cause you to exit ketosis will make your life a whole lot easier. Once you've determined this level, set this as your carb level in your macro calculation and add food as appropriate.

The best way of tracking your ketones is via a weekly average method. You could choose any one of the measuring techniques detailed previously and throughout the week consume the number of carbs you've set for yourself as per your macro calculation. If you find you're not able to maintain ketosis then you will need to decrease the carbs consumed.

On the other hand, if you're able to maintain ketosis, you could choose to increase your carb intake slightly, by say 10g per day, and look at the cumulative effect. This way, you can test your carb limit for ketosis and design your diet accordingly. It is not necessary for you to be at your carb limit but consuming a higher number of carbs could help you adjust to the keto diet better.

# WORKOUT TRACKING

There are a number of things you should be tracking when it comes to your workouts. Some of these are not strictly workout related but are important, nonetheless.

## *Weight*

Throughout the previous chapters, we've seen how tracking your weight is essential in determining your progress. To this effect, a weighing scale is a must buy along with the previously mentioned food weighing scale.

Always weigh yourself at the same time every day. So if you decide to weigh yourself right after waking up, on an empty stomach, always weight yourself at this time for as long as you're on the diet. You will find that your weight, on a day to day basis, will fluctuate. A lot of this has to do with water weight and other miscellaneous items that cause water retention or excretion.

Therefore, when you compare your weights across weeks, always compare the average weight NOT the day to day weight numbers. If you find that your average weight per week is reducing at a rate of 1 pound per week, this is a good sign. Don't pay much heed to the daily numbers, remember it is the average that counts.

## *Waist Size*

You can track your other physical measurements, like chest/bust, biceps, neck and so on but tracking your waist size is extremely important. More than anything else, this indicates your level of fat loss.

Just like with your weight, measure this at the same time every day and pay attention to the weekly average number.

## *Exercise Weight*

When you head to the gym, you need to carry a log book with you. This log will have the exercises you intend on performing that session, the sets and reps and the weight you intend to lift for that exercise. If you're performing cardio, it needs to record the intended session length.

Once you actually perform the exercises, you check off each set and rep and log whether you were able to complete that task or not. This logging is extremely important in any strength training program since you'll be increasing the weight on a regular basis.

## *Calories Burned*

While this number is not strictly necessary, if you use a Fitbit or any other activity tracker, it is helpful to use them to track your heart rate and calories burned during your workouts.

This, in turn, will help you determine whether your BMR numbers, which you estimate your diet macros off of, are accurate or not.

These are the important metric that you should be tracking at a bare minimum. Remember to keep reviewing these on a weekly basis to confirm whether you are on track or not. Any counter indications mean you need to go back and recalculate your macros and adjust your portions.

Next, we will look at the various aspects of meal prep and how you can do this easily.

# CHAPTER 10:

# KETO MEAL PREP

Now that you understand how to incorporate exercise plans into your lifestyle along with tracking your stats, all that remains to be looked at is meal prep. This is an area most people let themselves down in due to inconsistency and due to generally overlooking this.

When sitting down to figure out your meals, you'll probably go online and search for recipes and pick the ones that sound the most enticing. While there's nothing wrong with this approach, what most people ignore are the ramifications for their shopping list and the demands on time most of these diverse recipes call for.

With this in mind, let's now look at how to go about prepping your meals so that you don't have to sacrifice on taste and use your time in the most efficient manner possible.

# KETO STAPLES

The success or failure of any diet regime depends on how consistently you can enforce it. Following a diet is not about restricting yourself or saying "I can't eat this". Instead, it is looking at all the things you CAN do and reducing that list of things to the most repeatable and easy ones for you to follow.

You can look at various cookbooks and online recipes and come up with any number of recipes, all of which will be undoubtedly delicious. However, if these recipes require you to cook each and every one of them, every single time, you probably are not spending your time wisely.

If you have the time and inclination to cook then, of course, there's no problem. However, for most of us, work and other demands take up a significant amount of time. The best course of action is to reduce the diet to a few staples and mix these with a few rotating cast members, so to speak. The staples vegans need to stock up on are pretty self-explanatory since the majority of these are plant sourced. Generally speaking, there isn't anything special vegans need to do beyond prepare alternate protein sources.

This way your meal prep is reduced to a few minutes at the most and will involve either reheating or putting together your meal. So what are some of these staples?

## *Salad Greens*

Salads are simple and straightforward to prepare. Chop up your favorite veggies and toss them into a bowl and let them mix together. It's always a good idea to mix a big batch of salad greens together and store it in your fridge for further use. Salads by themselves are not very calorie dense and therefore, you need not worry about getting your portion size exactly right.

They're relatively easy to spice up as well! Toss in some onions or jalapenos to spice it up. Alternatively, you could put together a batch of homemade pico de gallo (tomatoes, onions, peppers, cilantro) and divide it into meal portions.

## *Baked Chicken Breast or Thighs*

Chicken is generally viewed as the most boring of meats and chicken breast is the least exciting bit of the bird. While all this is true, it is also, like most boring things, one of the healthiest proteins you can consume. You don't need to stand at the stove every single time to cook this. Simply bake a batch of them and reheat it for your meals portion-wise.

Baking, you will find, is one of the best ways to reduce your time in the kitchen and still have tasty meals ready to go. You could bake pretty much anything, including your vegetables or other meat. It is recommended to limit your red meat intake due to the previously mentioned saturated fat content in them. Once a week is perfectly fine though. If you're younger, say below the age of 25, then you can increase this pretty safely.

Chicken is an especially good option since it doesn't tend to lose its flavor when reheated, unlike other meat and fish. Turkey, for example, will often dry out easily when reheating and you might as well eat leather than eat reheated steak. Pairing your chicken breast with salads is an easy meal option.

Chicken thighs contain a higher amount of saturated fat and are tastier than chicken breast cuts. It's perfectly fine to consume chicken thighs as long as you minimize your consumption of them. In other words, instead of eating them every day, consume them as much as you would red meat.

### *Keto Snacks*

The snacks are perhaps the best bit about the keto diet. Given the abundance of fat the diet calls for, a whole world of possibilities opens up. You could go wild with bacon wrapped snacks and other exotic options but for consistency's sake, and if you don't have too much time to cook and prep your meals, a few staples will serve you well.

Dark chocolate and peanut butter along with some fatty nuts and dry fruits will fill you up more often than not. You can choose to combine these ingredients in any way possible. This is especially satisfying if you happen to have a sweet tooth. A dessert of peanut butter mixed with dark chocolate topped with whipped cream can rival anything a fancy restaurant has to offer.

## *Keto Bread and Tortillas*

One of the things most people struggle to get used to is the lack of grains in the keto diet. Most of us are used to eating rice or wheat in some form or another and find it difficult to feel full on just a salad.

With this in mind, it's a great idea to whip up a batch of keto bread or tortillas. These are made with coconut flour and you can find the recipes for the online quite easily. Store these away and you can now make pretty much anything from quesadillas to sandwiches to even pancakes for breakfast!

For those who prefer rice, whipping up a batch of keto rice, that is dehydrated cauliflower rice, is a good option. You should be careful with the portion sizes though since it could put you over your carb limits pretty easily.

The recipes for all of these are easily available if you search online or in any good ketogenic recipe books.

## *Eggs*

When in doubt, have some eggs. Don't feel like cooking anything? Have some eggs. Meal feels a bit light? Feeling hungrier than usual? Have some eggs.

Eggs are an excellent source of fat and protein. Make sure you eat the yolk along with the whites. While it is true that the yolk will have a negative effect on your cholesterol levels, with proper exercise, as you will be doing, this risk is minimized so eat the whole egg.

## *Cheese*

The previous section on eggs could be repeated word for word when it comes to cheese. A word of caution though: You should pay attention to what sort of cheese you are consuming. These days, given the proliferation of processed food, you will find a lot of cheeses made from vegetable oil and not from milk. Needless to stay, do not consume these.

Stick to a few base kinds of cheese like parmesan, ricotta, cheddar, and mozzarella. These are high in protein and are tasty to boot. You can also try cream cheese but most of these are highly processed so minimize your intake of these. Cottage cheese or farmer's cheese are also great options along with feta, halloumi and other Mediterranean and Levantine cheeses. Just make sure these are deli cheeses and not your garden variety supermarket counter cheese.

A word on processing: We've looked at this before but it bears repeating. All cheese is "processed". There is, however, a big difference between chemical processing and the processing that occurs as a natural part of the fermenting process. When you read about processing it refers to the chemical and other processing that doesn't make sense. For example, who ever heard of cheese coming from vegetables? So why would you consume cheese made from vegetable fat?

### Sardines or Tuna

Tuna is an old favorite of bodybuilders everywhere. It also happens to taste disgustingly bad. With this in mind, you could switch to sardines or mackerel. Sardines are a great, cheap and easy option to cook and add to your salads. You could also add anchovies or other dried fish.

Always keep a can of tuna or sardines handy in case you run out of food or feel too tired to put together a full meal.

In addition to the above you also want to stock up your kitchen with the foods below:

- Nuts and seeds
- Nut butters
- Herbs
- Thyme

- Oregano

- Garlic powder

- Parsley

- Dill

- Salt and pepper

- Coconut flour

- Coconut Cream

- Healthy oils like

- Olive Oil (refer to earlier sections regarding pomace versus extra virgin)

- Coconut oil

- Sesame oil

- Baking powder

- Mayonnaise

## FOODS TO MINIMIZE

The foods below are fully allowed on the keto diet but most people tend to take this as a free license to binge on these. Watch your portions when consuming these foods and minimize them as much as possible.

## Heavy Cream

It's the easiest source of fat you can find and it's equally easy to dunk everything into a pot of cream. Go easy on this because the cream is the last thing you want to overeat.

## Bacon

Everybody's favorite food is fully allowed on the keto diet. Searching recipes online will yield you a large majority of bacon-based recipes and most people forget to limit their intake of it. Bacon is full of saturated fat so you should minimize your intake of it, even if a daily dose of bacon falls within your macros.

## Artificial Sweetener

Sugar is completely out on the keto diet so most people, especially those who drink a lot of coffee or tea, feel compelled to add artificial sweeteners to their drink. Again, these are not naturally occurring foods so you should be very careful in limiting your intake of these. Stevia and the like are processed foods so, in the short term, a little bitterness in your coffee will pay dividends over the long run.

## Red Meat

While delicious, red meat has a high amount of saturated fat and you should be minimizing this. While some amount of saturated fat is good for us, an excess is clearly bad. The answer, therefore, as we say in the chapter on nutrition basics, is to minimize red meat and not cut it out completely. Stick to the leaner cuts of meat and consume this once or twice a week and you'll be fine.

## DIET DESIGN

We've already looked at the major points of designing a diet. This involves determining your activity levels and then based on your BMR, you need to calculate your macros at a deficit, maintenance or an excess depending on your goals.

A good idea when designing a diet is to add in cheat meals once a week. This cheat meal is not a license to binge but it is a day when you can relax your calorie consumption limit and can maybe go over your carb limit just a bit. Moderation is the key to this and is a point most people forget.

Another important point to keep in mind is that all calorie counts you see on software and your BMR rates etc are all estimates. They are not accurate down to the final calorie. This is why it is essential for you to constantly monitor your weight on a weekly basis. If you've observed that your mean weight has been increasing, its not a reason to panic or to beat yourself up. Instead, simply cut your calorie consumption by 250 kcal and track from there on out. Similarly, if you're losing too much weight, that is greater than 1 pound per week, you're eating too less and increase your intake by 250 kcal.

So for example, if you are really craving a pizza, instead of eating a full medium sized pie, have just a slice. Take your time to really savor it. Remember, if your diet feels overly restrictive and is causing you a lot of stress to keep up with, it's probably not for you. The best diet is one that you can follow.

There will always be some restrictive feeling whenever you begin a new diet or are disciplining yourself. You should not confuse this feeling with one of stress. If even after a month of following a new diet regimen, you find yourself dreading meal time or are spending an inordinate amount of time thinking and worrying about what you're eating, then it's probably an indication that this diet is not for you.

If you're on the CKD, a cheat meal really isn't necessary since the diet itself is a compromise so do keep that in mind.

Above all else, remember the first principle of dieting: Always design something that is as repeatable as possible. This is why we've looked at staples and exercise regimes that are basic and can be implemented with the least amount of effort. Dieting and disciplining yourself is tough to begin with. You owe it to yourself to make this as smooth as possible.

## *Tools for Starting Meal Prep*

In addition to the staple foods listed above, you will need the following kitchen equipment to get up and running:

- Skillet

- Quality Knife

- Slow cooker or crockpot

- Parchment paper

- Baking dishes

- Food processor

Food weighing scale and other tracking equipment as listed in the previous chapter

Purchasing a quality cast iron skillet along with a good chef's knife will reduce your meal prep times and simply make your life a whole lot easier when it comes to preparing your meals. The skillet will come in handy when you need to quickly prepare some eggs or bacon. Generally speaking, to minimize your time spent in the kitchen (assuming this is what you want), baking and slow cooking are your best options. The best slow cooker would be an Instant Pot where you can simply throw everything in and let it work its magic.

Food processors will help you with preparing great tasting carb substitutes like cauliflower rice and in addition to this, you can also whip up some great options like seed butters, smoothies etc.

### Steps to Successful Prep

Prepping your meals successfully is a pretty straightforward task as evidenced by the list below:

Plan your meals a week in advance

- Plan cooking schedule (either cooked in advance of scratch)

- Shop

- Cook

**Step 1** is the most important of all. It is necessary when you're starting out to plan everything in advance since you'll be dealing with a lot of other adjustments when you adopt the keto diet.

Plan your breakfasts, lunches and dinners along with a staple few snacks like nuts and butters, you will consume. As mentioned previously, to make this easy, repeat as many meals as possible. When choosing recipes, you can go online and search for recipes which already have the macros listed in them and easily calculate your portions.

While this helps in the short term, over the longer term, it pays to reduce your ingredients for the week to a few staples and then decide on the recipes from there, based on how much you would like to eat them. Relying on someone else's calorie counts will only lead to laziness and that's the last thing you want.

**Step 2** is where you will decide when to cook your meals. Cook your meals in the easiest and most repeatable manner possible. While cooking in advance is tempting, its not a good idea to make your meals more than 2 days in advance. Storing cooked meals in the fridge will reduce the taste and in the case of red meat or chicken, change the texture of the meat and make it less tasty.

While convenience is important, don't follow it at the cost of making things hard on yourself. While out shopping, that is step 3, make sure to purchase quantities for the entire week. You can easily calculate this from step 1. Alternatively, you could work backwards from the quantity you would like to consume and design recipes around it. For example, if you prefer consuming 100 grams of chicken thighs everyday, purchase 1kg of thighs and store it in your freezer.

Prepping your meals and cooking them will take some adjusting to, especially if you're used to consuming foods from the center aisles of your department store (which is where all the processed foods are). Taking it slow and methodically mapping out each and every step is the key to success with this.

# CONCLUSION

The ketogenic diet is a wonderful way to lose fat or gain muscle or even to do both simultaneously. The diet's requirements are quite basic and easy to follow. Allied with the right exercise program, you will see guaranteed results.

Remember to always keep the basics of nutrition and exercise in mind as you go about implementing this in your life. A caloric deficit is necessary for you to lose weight and a caloric excess is for gaining weight. Always track how much you're eating and also track the various parameters we looked at in the chapter on tracking. It is the average numbers you want to pay attention to, not the day to day numbers which will fluctuate.

Depending on your goals you can choose to adopt the SKD, HPKD, CKD or TKD. While the TKD and HPKD are for slightly more experienced people, you can always adopt them after following the SKD or CKD. It is important to be aware of your goals right from the start, whether it is to lose fat or gain muscle or recompose the lean muscle mass versus fat your body. If you're not able to decide on what you need first, asking those around you or going with your gut feeling is usually the best option.

Keep your shelves stocked with some keto staples and you will make your life a lot easier when it comes to making meals, especially if you don't have the time or inclination to spend a lot of time in the kitchen. Prepare these in batches and them together and you'll have tasty and nutritious meals ready in no time.

Revisiting the first few chapters regarding the basics of nutrition and exercise will do you a world of good. Initially, it will seem like a lot but keep at it and you will reap the rewards!

Thank you very much, once again, for purchasing this book. If you feel you've learned something useful and if this book has helped you take a step towards your goals, please do leave a review, it is much appreciated!

# BIBLIOGRAPHY

Chapter 1

1: Nutrition. (2019). Retrieved from https://www.who.int/topics/nutrition/en/

2: Water: How much should you drink every day?. (2019). Retrieved from https://www.mayoclinic.org/healthy-lifestyle/nutrition-and-healthy-eating/in-depth/water/art-20044256

Chapter 2

1: Mandal, A. (2019). History of the Ketogenic Diet. Retrieved from https://www.news-medical.net/health/History-of-the-Ketogenic-Diet.aspx

2: Foster, G., Wyatt, H., Hill, J., McGuckin, B., Brill, C., & Mohammed, B. et al. (2003). A Randomized Trial of a Low-Carbohydrate Diet for Obesity. New England Journal Of

Medicine, 348(21), 2082-2090. doi: 10.1056/nejmoa022207

3: Brehm, B., Seeley, R., Daniels, S., & D'Alessio, D. (2003). A Randomized Trial Comparing a Very Low Carbohydrate Diet and a Calorie-Restricted Low Fat Diet on Body Weight and Cardiovascular Risk Factors in Healthy Women. The Journal Of Clinical Endocrinology & Metabolism, 88(4), 1617-1623. doi: 10.1210/jc.2002-021480

4: Daly, M., Paisey, R., Paisey, R., Millward, B., Eccles, C., & Williams, K. et al. (2006). Short-term effects of severe dietary carbohydrate-restriction advice in Type 2 diabetes-a randomized controlled trial. Diabetic Medicine, 23(1), 15-20. doi: 10.1111/j.1464-5491.2005.01760.x

5: Gasior, M., Rogawski, M. A., & Hartman, A. L. (2006). Neuroprotective and disease-modifying effects of the ketogenic diet. Behavioral Pharmacology, 17(5-6), 431-9.

6, 7: Zhou, W., Mukherjee, P., Kiebish, M. A., Markis, W. T., Mantis, J. G., & Seyfried, T. N. (2007). The calorically restricted ketogenic diet, an effective alternative therapy for malignant brain cancer. Nutrition & Metabolism, 4, 5. doi:10.1186/1743-7075-4-5

8: Paoli, A., Grimaldi, K., Toniolo, L., Canato, M., Bianco, A., & Fratter, A. (2012). Nutrition and Acne: Therapeutic Potential of Ketogenic Diets. Skin Pharmacology And

Physiology, 25(3), 111-117. doi: 10.1159/000336404

Chapter 3

1: Cronkleton, E., & Sullivan, D. (2019). What Happens If You Eat Too Much Protein?. Retrieved from https://www.healthline.com/health/too-much-protein#recommended-daily-protein

Chapter 5

1, 2: McCall, P. (2019). 7 Things to Know About Excess Post-exercise Oxygen Consumption (EPOC). Retrieved from **HTTPS://WWW.ACEFITNESS.ORG/EDUCATION-AND-RESOURCES/PROFESSIONAL/EXPERT-ARTICLES/5008/7-THINGS-TO-KNOW-ABOUT-EXCESS-POST-EXERCISE-OXYGEN-CONSUMPTION-EPOC**

3: Veracity, D. (2019). Bone density sharply enhanced by weight training, even in the elderly. Retrieved from **HTTPS://WWW.NATURALNEWS.COM/010528_BONE_DENSITY_MINERAL.HTML**

4: Long-term weight training may benefit Parkinson's disease patients. (2019). Retrieved from **HTTPS://WWW.NEWS-MEDICAL.NET/NEWS/20120217/LONG-TERM-**

# WEIGHT-TRAINING-MAY-BENEFIT-PARKINSONS-DISEASE-PATIENTS.ASPX

5: Schmitz, K., Ahmed, R., Troxel, A., Cheville, A., Smith, R., & Lewis-Grant, L. et al. (2009). Weight Lifting in Women with Breast-Cancer–Related Lymphedema. New England Journal Of Medicine, 361(7), 664-673. doi: 10.1056/nejmoa0810118

6: Häkkinen A, Häkkinen K, Hannonen P, et al. Strength training induced adaptations in neuromuscular function of premenopausal women with fibromyalgia: comparison with healthy women. Annals of the Rheumatic Diseases 2001;60:21-26.

7: De Backer, I., Van Breda, E., Vreugdenhil, A., Nijziel, M., Kester, A., & Schep, G. (2007). High-intensity strength training improves quality of life in cancer survivors. Acta Oncologica, 46(8), 1143-1151. doi: 10.1080/02841860701418838

# Intermittent Fasting for Women 30-Day Challenge

Complete Weight Loss Guide for Women: Burn Fat, Slim Down, and Heal Your Body

# INTRODUCTION

Imagine this: you are on a beach in Miami, wearing your floral wrap-around dress and a two-piece swimsuit underneath. You feel confident as ever; the wind in your face, the warm water splashes on your legs. It feels so real to finally feel sexy. You feel like everybody has been staring at you the whole time but not in a negative way. It merely feels as if they are in awe of your beauty and body. You feel young and beautiful; it is like you can conquer the world once again with your profound body.

This time, you remember what it feels to be a bullied teenager in high school. Think of the names that the bullies used to yell at you over and over again. Whale! Pig! Ugly! It does not seem to add much, but it hurts more than they know. People saw you as a source of traffic – a nuisance in society - because of your weight. I mean, you cannot ride the bus without experiencing the judging stares, telling you that your body covers two seats and that it is better if you stand up for the benefit of others than to remain sitting.

Sometimes, you feel embarrassed to ask for an extra scoop of ice cream or an extra bowl of salad without the customers' and waiters' eyes trained on you as well. It feels so sad to live the life of an overweight teenager. It seems like every day is a trial that you outwait until you get home and rest, only to repeat the same cycle the next day.

There are many reasons why a woman grows stout. One of them is aging. But this should not make you stop striving to have the sexy body that you deserve. Imagine still getting to wear your two-piece at the age of 40. People would ask, "How old are you?" They would not believe their eyes even when you tell them that you are already 45 years old. With the body of a superstar, you will be mistaken as someone in your early 20s. Trust me when I say that you can still regain that super-hot body of yours.

Giving birth is the most magical event of all time. However, it has a lot of physical effects on the mother, especially without exercise and proper diet. Most moms let themselves go and give no regard to their bodies after birth. But sooner than later, they start to regret the extra pounds that they have gained from being a full-time mother. If you are having the same problems, you have come to the right place. Who said you cannot be sexy again in a matter of 30 days? YOU CAN, AND YOU WILL! Let me guide you through it step by step.

If you are afraid that people will judge you by having this book, don't be! There are millions of women out there who would give anything to be led on the road to weight loss by hand. Better yet, be proud that you are doing something for yourself to achieve a goal and feel young, beautiful, and sexy from the inside and out.

## THE HISTORY OF FASTING AND WEIGHT LOSS

Our ancestors have started fasting as early as the 3rd century BC when the Greeks regarded stoutness as a form of physical abnormality – a result of corruption, sloth, and greed. This was the reason why their scientists such as Hippocrates recommended the balance between extremities, introducing a smooth and sensible lifestyle that could help the people get back in shape. Hippocrates, being the father of medicine, focused his energy and research in highlighting the importance of understanding the health of the patient, the independence and health of mind, the harmony deep within the individual, and the social and natural environments he lives in. He constituted the saying that goes, "A healthy mind in a healthy body", which is one of the main principles of the Hippocratic philosophy. He was the first person to believe that diseases were not brought at all by demons and spirits. Rather, they were brought by either physical deprivation or gluttony. He also found that people can cope with these illnesses through a balanced diet, rest, and healthy physical activities.

It was Hippocrates who proposed the relationship between the body and the mind. An ill body could cause an ill mind, and vice versa. He claimed in his research that a person's beliefs, ideas, thought, and feelings, came from the brain, not the heart, and it had a significant effect to the physiological aspect of a person. Obviously so, whenever we are depressed, we are less inclined to work and concentrate. We feel as if every part of our body hurts as much as our heart. But if we feel happy, we are more energetic and motivated to get things done and go through a whole day no matter how hard it is. This theory of the Father of Medicine can be quite useful in our journey towards weight loss. Nevertheless, we will get more into that later.

In a more specific sense, fasting has its own roots that dates back to Hippocrates as well. Over the years, the method has been a time-tested tradition. It is not only used for weight loss but also for improving concentration, extending human life, preventing Alzheimer's disease, increasing insulin resistance, and even slowing down the aging process. The theory of fasting comes from the idea that lowering the insulin levels promote weight gain. The problem is that all foods significantly increase the levels of insulin in the body. So, the only way to lose weight effectively is to abstain from food. Hence, the term 'fasting' was born.

According to experts, one of the most common mistakes done by people who try to lose weight is searching for an all-exotic food variety that can make them lose weight. Others resort to products that are meant for slimming, which they do not know are harmful to the body and might cause more trouble than good when taken. Some specialists have come up with the conclusion that the only way to significantly feel weight loss is through old and proven methods like fasting.

You would be surprised to know who initiated the revolution towards fasting. After all, it was no other than Hippocrates of Cos. He was the one who started the consumption of apple cider vinegar to lose weight. According to one of his principles, "To eat when you are sick is to feed your illness." This was later echoed by the Greek writer and historian named Plutarch who claimed, "Instead of using a medicine, better fast today." Other researchers claimed that even Plato and his student Aristotle were both advocates of the concept of fasting. Scientists from ancient Greece believed that this method was known as the "physician within." It is the instinct that makes not only humans but also animals anorexic when they get sick. This can be observed in modern times when there is a significant decline in appetite whenever a person is ill. Apparently, there is an internal rationale for feeling that way, and it should not be ignored. Most of us are forced to take in chunks of food even when we have no appetite. Our doctors and parents would urge us to eat a significant amount of food when we get sick. "Eat your food so that you can take your medicine" - this is the most common sentence we hear whenever we acquire an illness. However, what if we start to listen to our forefathers and believe we merely feed the virus in our body when we eat? Or, even if we do, we should resort to healthy foods and count the calories much like what Lulu Peters and William Banting had proposed. Our bodies have their own antibacterial properties. Can't you see that the main reason why viruses and bacteria get stronger every day is because of the countless breakthroughs and innovation in medicine?

Let us take a look at the opinions of other intellectual giants. The founder of toxicology, Philip Paracelsus, was also a great supporter of fasting. He is one of the three founders of modern Western medicine along with Hippocrates and Galen, who wrote that fasting is the greatest remedy. This idea was supported by Benjamin Franklin, one of America's founding fathers, who said that the best of all medicines is resting and fasting. In a religious perspective, did you know that Jesus Christ, Buddha, and Muhammed shared the same belief regarding the benefits of fasting? According to their wisdom, the practice aids in cleansing and purification the body. In Buddhism, food is only consumed in the morning, and the followers do not eat anything for the rest of the day.

Hence, the first meal in the morning is known as breakfast. Meaning, "to break the fasting." For Muslims, it is an important part of tradition to fast from sunrise to sunset during Ramadan, their holy month. The Prophet Muhammad encouraged people to skip meals on Mondays and Thursdays every week as well. As you can see, fasting indeed withstood the hands of time. Until now, it is recognized as one of the most effective ways to stay healthy.

However, whenever some individuals think about the process of fasting, they become skeptic towards its effects on the human body. Other assume that the practice means starvation and self-torture. To set things straight, fasting is way too different from starvation. First and foremost, when you say the latter, it entails an involuntary absence of food, which is often the effect of poverty or lack of resources. The former term, meanwhile, refers to voluntary abstinence for physical, spiritual, and mental purposes. When you fast, you choose when and what to eat. These two words should not be mistaken with each other because they are not the same. One of the main reasons why I am writing this book is to enlighten people about the advantages of fasting and to break the stigma that many have associated with this golden process.

# TYPES OF FASTING

There are several fasting methods out there. Although some of them might not be as famous as intermittent fasting, it is best to have an idea about the others for the sake of having choices in the long run. Who knows, maybe after you have successfully reached your ideal body structure, you can try other practices and discover more than what meets the eye.

### *Occasional Short Fasts*

This type of fasting is the starting point for most people. This does not follow a consistent schedule; it merely constitutes an occasional fast for six, 12 or 24 hours. There is not much commitment to this technique, though, there is no guarantee that it will work. See, some people indeed engage in fasting. The problem is, when it is time for them to eat, they consume food voraciously, forgetting what they have just done before that and why.

### *Intermittent Fasting*

Intermittent fasting, as mentioned earlier, is one of the most effective ways of fasting because it requires commitment and a whole new level of discipline. This method is defined as a regular act of abstinence. For example, you skip meals for one, two or three days a week. In the succeeding chapters, we will be discussing the power and practices related to intermittent fasting. From what some experts have said, after all, it is a form of partial fasting that helps you develop a dietary routine. Apart from the fact that it helps you control your eating habits, it can also allow you to do other activities, such as sports and hobbies.

### *Longer Fasts*

This is by one of the most difficult kinds of fasting because it entails that you will abstain from eating for three days to one week. It is far more difficult than intermittent fasting and requires times ten of commitment and discipline. Plus, most people who start fasting with this technique end up giving up because they cannot endure the hunger, pain, and discomfort that come with longer fasts.

### *Extended Fasting*

Extended fasting is another challenging form of fasting since it means that you will extend a scheduled fast for two hours or more. Imagine going beyond a three-day fast. Imagine the discipline and self-control needed for such ordeal. Much like longer fasts, you need to have an experience with this method already and be able to master your thoughts. Otherwise, you might be doing more harm than good to your body.

## *Open-Ended Fasts*

An open-ended fast is one of the most common fasting techniques of all time. When you do it, you can break your commitment to the method after reaching your goals. Extended fasts and intermittent fasting are a couple of its examples. Then, you may resort to occasional fasting to maintain your health and physical appearance.

## *Occasional or Longer Group Fasting*

There are organizations that facilitate occasional group fasting. This can help you stay on track towards a successful fast. There is a leader to monitor your achievements every day, every week, and every month. Whenever you feel sad or down about not being able to live life to the fullest, you can open up to your superiors to gain uplifting advices to get you to keep on fasting.

# CHAPTER 1:

## INTERMITTENT FASTING FOR WOMEN

If you are looking for the best way to lose weight in just 30 days, you have come to the right place! In this book, I am not only teaching you how to fast intermittently, but I am also incorporating some methods of motivation and self-discipline. As our father of medicine, Hippocrates, has theorized, there is a back-and-forth connection between the body and mind. Without a proper mindset, intermittent fasting will not be as effective as you want it to be, regardless of how long you do it.

The answer to your prayers does not lie on the new diets that you see on the web. You cannot depend on the dietary supplements in the stores either. You see, even if you try it all, nothing can make you lose weight if you have no idea about the power of fasting. Furthermore, none of those methods have withstood the test of time as much as fasting has. Even when you adopt one of the most famous weight-loss methods out there, how sure are you that you will not develop any illness in the future because of it? How can you tell with certainty that you will not revert to your old body once you stop following the fad?

Of course, to sell their products, the creators of new diets and dietary supplements will claim that they are "guaranteed safe and effective." However, after 10 or 20 years of usage, who can ensure that you will not contract a chronic disease due to the chemicals and substances that are in such products?

The so-called "treatments" mentioned above have not been proven effective in a matter of centuries. The people who have employed fasting as a method of weight loss, on the other hand, have reported to be more alert and energetic in their daily activities. Several celebrities do intermittent fasting as well to maintain their bodies and maintain a healthy lifestyle. Some of the female personalities who do so include Beyoncé, Jennifer Lopez, Selena Gomez, Nicole Kidman, and Miranda Kerr. For the men, we have Benedict Cumberbatch, Hugh Jackman, Terry Crews, and Chris Hemsworth. If you are wondering how they get the energy to accomplish all of their activities in Hollywood, it must have something to do with fasting intermittently.

Other famous people such as Kourtney Kardashian, Moby, Molly Sims, Chris Pratt, and Paul Krugman also swear to intermittent fasting. John Kane, who experimented on the practice, claimed that ever since he started employing the method, he had been brighter, sharper, and happier than ever in life. He said that it could wake people up and hype up the energy. Although he did not follow any standard plan of fasting, he benefited from it and was contented with the results.

As easy as it may seem not to eat, some individuals cannot stick to intermittent fasting. The main reason is lack of discipline and motivation. For people who have been used to a voracious lifestyle, after all, it is hard for them to say no when they see a muffin, cake, junk food, or other enticing stuff in the corner or the ref. Because of their frustration, they get stressed out, depressed, anxious, and apprehended, causing them to binge-eat and gain weight even more. The problem with these individuals is not their food intake. Instead, it is their mindset towards the methods of weight loss. This is the main reason why we need to discuss several ways to train your mind before fasting in the following chapters.

# INTERMITTENT FASTING

The popularity of intermittent fasting among countries is spreading like a wildfire in this era. From the term itself, intermittent fasting (IF) is a pattern of eating and not eating during a specific period. The process involves limiting your caloric intake in certain days or weeks by merely allowing you to consume foods in a few hours daily. For example, you may eat breakfast, but you cannot any food for the rest of the day. Others employ time as their signal to eat. Some people only eat at 7 in the morning and in the evening without consuming anything in between.

Though its main cause of fame is its relation to weight loss, intermittent fasting was first used for disease prevention and longevity. Its ability to help you lose weight is just a bonus. Studies have shown that when food is restricted from lab rats and other species such as mice, hamsters, and yeast, this can extend their lifespan by a significant amount of time. As mentioned earlier, this procedure has also supported the theory of Paracelsus and Hippocrates when they advise people not to eat when they are sick. Modern research has found that bad cells are being killed in the process of fasting, too, so it seems to enhance the body's ability to counteract foreign bodies.

In the year 2017, researchers have worked together to know whether fasting can reduce the onset of diabetes, cancer, and cardiovascular diseases. In this study, they have randomized 100 samples into two groups for three months. The first group was allowed to eat anything they want, and the latter group fasted for days each month. After the experimentation, the researchers have gathered that fasting can really improve someone's health. It caused weight loss, lowered blood pressure, and decreased the genetic marker for cancer, the IGF–1. However, there were a lot of people who gave up in the fasting phase, which led them to believe that fasting is a difficult but effective method. Apart from this conclusion, though, there are other surprising benefits of intermittent fasting to human beings.

If you aim to reach your maximum height potential, consider fasting as a way to boost your human growth hormone (HGH). The practice makes it skyrocket in your body and allows you to grow taller and leaner as time goes by. The levels of insulin can also normalize through fasting by making stored body fat more accessible for expending or burning. Researches have also found that intermittent fasting can contribute to cellular repair - a process that gets rid of dead cells and dysfunctional proteins that build up inside human cells. It can also increase your metabolic rate by 3.6% to 14%, thus deeming it the most powerful tool for weight loss. In a study conducted in 2016, people who employed intermittent fasting as a weight-loss remedy showed a significant rate of 3% to 8% weight reduction in 3 - 24 weeks' time. The same researchers also gathered that people could reduce their waistline by 4% to 7% through intermittent fasting.

In a more serious note, intermittent fasting also prevents inflammation in the body, which is the key indicator of chronic diseases. Hippocrates and John Kane were right by saying that this method could improve your alertness and energy. Furthermore, studies show that the practice does not only make you lose weight but also promote brain health and prevent Alzheimer's disease. Other researchers have revealed that intermittent fasting can detoxify the body. It helps you get rid of harmful chemicals and substances that may cause diseases. In turn, it promotes cell regeneration as early as 2-4 days since following the method. From the data gathered, intermittent fasting can aid in boosting the immune system as well, protecting the body and its cells from foreign entities, as well as cellular damage that's due to external factors like UV rays and chemotherapy.

### *Who Should Not Fast?*

It is no secret that not all individuals are allowed to fast. People with eating disorders and depression, for instance, should not try fasting at all because it worsens their condition and might cause serious damages to the body. We have discussed at the beginning of the chapter how serotonin, being the happy hormone, works against depression. It is needed to avert the effects of sadness and frustration, and it can only be acquired through food intake. Depressed patients are required to eat three times a day with snacks in between to promote the secretion of serotonin, which usually comes from the breakdown of food into sugar. Without ample food in the body, the person stays depressed and may even start entertaining suicidal thoughts.

Anorexia nervosa patients should not be allowed to fast as well. This eating disorder is characterized by excessive weight loss or lack of sufficient weight gain. It inhibits an individual from maintaining an appropriate weight, height, and stature for a specific age. Moreover, people with anorexia nervosa have a distorted body image. They see themselves as overweight even when they no longer have any fat to burn, and they appear all skin and bones to normal folks. This disorder can affect all ages, though it usually starts in adolescence when people - especially women - seek a sense of belonging in groups. When a lady has anorexia, for instance, she will not eat and probably starve herself to look good in her own eyes. She tends to deny her hunger when others ask why she won't eat; even when she does pick up the fork and spoon, she will take an excessive amount of laxatives to expel the calories taken. If not, the lady might force herself to regurgitate all the food and exercise extraneously just to "get in shape." Anorexia nervosa is one of the scariest eating disorders because it can lead to severe conditions, such as stomach cancer, ulcer, and death. We have even gathered that the "anything goes" mentality that some experts permit during the feeding state can make someone overeat and create guilt, shame, and other problems that can only become worse over time. For someone with emotional or psychological eating disorders, intermittent fasting can, therefore, become a convenient crutch to amplify such issues.

Furthermore, fasting can be helpful for individuals dealing with gut issues, stress, and anxiety. When you have gastroesophageal reflux disorder (GERD), a form of a stomach illness, fasting is not recommended either. This illness is characterized by heartburn or acid indigestion since the stomach does not have enough food to churn.

The problem is, some experts say that fasting can amplify anxiety and stress in certain individuals. Apparently, once folks with these conditions fast, they tend to be "hangry" when there is an imbalance of cortisol in the body. They become temperamental, irritable, and anxious, thus leaving them either aggressive or unproductive throughout the day. If you notice such symptoms in yourself, consult your doctor or psychiatrist before you employ fasting as a weight-loss remedy.

Pregnant and breastfeeding mothers should not be allowed to fast as well. You will need every nutrient you can get to help your child develop in the womb. Also, when you are underweight and undernourished, you no longer need to fast. Instead, you need to do the opposite and eat as many foods as you can to compensate for your insufficient weight. When you are trying to conceive children, maintain a healthy diet, but avoid fasting. This can cause hormonal imbalance, which makes conception a more difficult process.

Having amenorrhea is also an indication for women that fasting is not for you. This condition is characterized by the absence of menstruation for months at a time. When you have an irregular cycle, it is possible that you are not using enough subcutaneous fat as energy during menstruation. You may lack in nutrients needed for the blood to circulate properly in your body as well, thus throwing your hormones and bodily chemicals out of balance. One of the most common causes of amenorrhea is pregnancy. So, when you have a missed period, check for any signs of pregnancy and do not fast. Instead, consume many fruits, vegetables, and every nutritious food in the book, including water.

Also, when you are under medications for certain illnesses, such as diabetes and anemia, make sure that you have your physician's go signal before fasting. There are instances when medicines work poorly without the assistance of food to absorb the substances.

## Disadvantages of Fasting

Much like any other weight-loss method, there are also disadvantages of intermittent fasting that we should not ignore. From the experiments and observations conducted by doctors, they have found that fasting can cause dehydration to people because the body does not get enough food. Fasting is also known to increase stress and disrupt sleep as it aids in the secretion of cortisol in the body. If you do not get enough food, you may become more irritable and agitated. It can cause headache, stomach ache, and muscle pain, especially during hard work. Nausea can also be a common effect of fasting because of the lack of sugar in the body. It is true the practice can lower blood pressure, too; however, excessive fasting can do that at a dangerous rate. Scientists and experts have also found that the method contributes to heartburn and acidity because of the unexpended stomach acids.

## Myths about Intermittent Fasting

1. It Is Dangerous to Your Health.

When people think about fasting, they roll their eyes and assume that it will be bad for your health. They will even dissuade you from doing it because these individuals believe that it can do more harm than good to you. What they do not understand is the effects and science of doing intermittent fasting as you go along. As long as you have been given permission to do so, I do not see why you cannot try it.

## 2. You Should Not Drink Liquids When Fasting.

This is one of the reasons why people remain skeptic about the powers of intermittent fasting. In reality, you can drink coffee, green tea, and water in between your fast breaks to avoid ulcer and other gut-related illnesses.

## 3. Skipping Breakfast Is Unhealthy.

There is a stigma that says people who skip breakfast have unhealthy lifestyles. Many folks fast for various reasons, not just to lose weight. Just look at the health benefits that intermittent fasting can bring to your body. If you choose a fasting schedule that requires you to skip breakfast, it should not be a problem. Others do that all the time even if they are not fasting. They prefer having a meal in between instead, which you might know more of as 'brunch.'

## 4. You Cannot Take Supplements While Fasting.

Food supplements are excellent sources of vitamins and minerals that the body requires. When you are employing intermittent fasting as a means of living healthily, it is perfectly okay to take them while following the IF method.

## 5. Fasting Can Cause Muscle Loss.

Every weight-loss method has this side effect, and intermittent fasting is not any different. Nevertheless, you can counter it by taking high levels of protein and maintaining regular exercise even when you are fasting to promote muscle building.

## 6. Children Can Fast, Too.

Kids are not allowed to fast at all. Even if your child is obese or overweight, he or she should not be subjected to intermittent fasting. To help them lose weight, it is important to promote another technique, such as the fruit diet, water cleansing, regular exercise, and reduction of caloric intake in every meal.

# CHAPTER 2:

# SCIENCE BEHIND

# INTERMITTENT FASTING

Hippocrates and his colleagues did not develop the concept of fasting by using their instinct or opinions. It took them years of experimentation, as well as observing individuals who experienced it. They even tried fasting themselves to see and feel its effects within the human body.

In this chapter, I will be discussing how fasting works. To be specific, how does the method affect the cells? What does it do to promote its health benefits? Understanding the science behind this concept is a vital tool to garner an idea on how it can useful for you. I am sure you do not want to be shocked by the sudden changes it can bring as you continue to fast intermittently. We have also discussed in the previous chapters that fasting is not for everyone. Knowing what it should feel like now can help you understand if it is right for you or not. You also need to know if you are doing it properly or not.

Every minute of every day, our body needs energy. Whether we are resting, procrastinating or engaging in strenuous work, we need sugar to kickstart our organs and keep our blood flowing efficiently in our veins. The form of sugar we need in our body to be converted into energy is called carbohydrates, which are found in grains, dairy products, fruits, vegetables, beans, concessionaires, and others. Our muscles and liver secrete glucose to our bloodstream, especially when the body is performing an activity. Without it, you can become weaker and might not be able to accomplish any task for the day.

When a person engages in fasting, this whole process changes. After about eight hours of food abstinence, the liver will have used up all its glucose reserves up to the last drop. When this happens, the body goes into a state called gluconeogenesis, which switches the body into fasting mode. In this phase, you increase the number of calories that you burn. Without the glucose secreted by the liver, it generates its own form of energy using the fats inside the body, thus promoting weight loss. However, fasting becomes starvation when there are no more fats to use up. This causes dangerous effects on the body; that's why you need to break this fast on a timely yet efficient schedule. Without any fat to burn, your metabolism starts to slow down, and you will start to burn muscles for energy, so your muscle mass will reduce and put the body in a more hazardous state.

## TYPES OF INTERMITTENT FASTING

It is imperative to take fasting as more than a mere hobby. Without proper guidance and schedule of meals, you might be putting your body on grave danger. Intermittent fasting is not only about the concept of food abstinence. There are specific guidelines to follow to get more benefits. Luckily, experts have created several methods for successful intermittent fasting. These schedules will help you assess what schedule of fasting and eating is suitable for your body. In this segment, I will be discussing 15 types of intermittent fasting to choose from. It is advised to start from the basic methods to gain experience as you go along with the process.

1. 24-Hour Fasting

From the name itself, this method of intermittent fasting allows you to fast for 24 hours before having a meal. However, for people who are not yet as experienced in fasting, this is not advisable. The only time you should engage in 24-hour fasting is when you have finally established your body and mind to longer fasts. Without ample experience in fasting, you might be doing more harm than good to your body, especially when it is not used to abstaining from food at this particular amount of time. In this process, you can even eat at the 23rd hour and take in food for one hour to impose a higher calorie deficit.

## 2. 16/8 Intermittent Fasting

This type of fasting has been popularized by Martin Borkhan of Leangains. It optimizes weight loss with heavy and strenuous exercise. The concept is simple: you abstain from food for 16 hours and then eat within 8 hours. The number of meals you have for the day or week is not relevant in this kind of intermittent fasting. For this method, most people choose to skip breakfast and eat around noon. Therefore, they have an exact 16 hours from dinner until noon before they can eat at a time frame of exactly 8 hours. Others stop eating at around 8 P.M. and resume eating from 12 P.M. the next day until 7 P.M. For them, it is the perfect time to fast - and the easiest one at that. I, on the other hand, stop eating at around 6 P.M. onwards and resume eating at 10 A.M. the next day. When I have so much work to do, I get hungry in the morning. So, instead of waiting at 12 P.M., I eat at 10 A.M.

## 3. The Warrior Diet

This originated from the ancient four years like the Spartans in Rome who would stay physically active the entire day and only eat at night. During daylight, they were not allowed to eat because they were too preoccupied in building barracks and fortresses, including equipment for their beloved country. The only thing that helped them acquire the energy they needed for strength and stamina was beer, which was totally permitted for intermittent fasting. Evening was the only time they were allowed to eat huge portions of foods such as stew, meat, bread, and other varieties.

## 4. OMAD

OMAD is more popularly known as One Meal a Day. I am sure that most of you might have heard the saying, "An apple a day keeps the doctor away." But according to our father of medicine, Hippocrates, fasting is the best way to heal the body from illnesses. Hence, in this method, you will be fasting for about 21 to 23 hours and can merely eat for 1 to 3 hours. It doesn't matter which meal you eat as long as you are comfortable with the timeframe. If you have work to do in the morning, it is preferable to eat during breakfast and skip your meals until the next day. There are others who skip their breakfast and dinner and only eat lunch or brunch, whichever they see fit. Researchers believe that the method of eating once a day is ideal for losing fat but not for muscle growth. Apparently, fasting for 21 hours and above is enough to convert muscles into energy, which can be detrimental to other people.

## 5. 36-Hour Fasting

In earlier times, people can go for days without eating food. Nowadays, most doctors will not prescribe it. A person cannot even skip breakfast sometimes, let alone a snack during breaktime. Experts, however, have proven that fasting for over 24 hours can do wonders to the body. They have gathered that the longer you stay fasted and experience energy deprivation, the body is forced to trigger its longevity pathway to help mobilize fast, boost stem cells, and recycle worn-out cells. According to some studies, it takes at least one day to see significant effects of autophagy. But this process can be sped up by eating a low-carb diet before starting to fast and exercising on an empty stomach. Researchers also recommend using herbal teas to stimulate the process of autophagy. Unfortunately, such methods are not yet applicable for intermittent fasting enthusiasts. As mentioned a while back, it takes courage, determination, commitment, and self-discipline to accomplish this specific practice.

Before we move on to the next type of intermittent fasting, let us first discuss what autophagy is and what it means to the body. This is an internal process that aids in the destruction of dysfunctional cells. The term autophagy literally means "to eat itself." However, there is nothing to be alarmed about because it maintains homeostasis in the body by allowing the detoxification of bad substances to make way for cell regeneration. The purpose of autophagy is to balance the manufacture of cellular components and destroy the damaged cells and dysfunctional organelles. It may have seemed like a dangerous concept at first, it is needed by the body for healthier organs and skin.

## 6. 48-Hour Fasting

The 48-hour fasting is one of the most difficult forms of intermittent fasting. Once you've made it past the 36th hour, you can try this as well. A highly challenging part of this type of fasting is the adaptation phase in which the body is forced to cope with the changes it comes with. However, once you get used to the method, it will be easier to engage in more forms of fasting than the easiest ones. According to people who have experienced 48-hour fasting, they have reached ketosis faster, a state that activates autophagy. You will develop the ability to suppress hunger, feel mentally clear, and have a bit more energy and focus when you do so.

Like we said in the previous chapters, intermittent fasting can be a form of extended fasting when you chooses to increase the time of food abstinence. Still, based on a research, fasting up to the 24-hour mark is the most difficult battle to accomplish. If you want to commit this kind of strategy in the long run, you should train your mind and body to adjust to the physiological effects of extended fasting.

## 7. Extended Fasting

If you are wondering if there's something more exhausting than the 48-hour fasting, there is a method called extended fasting that can last for 3 to 7 days. According to several experiments, 72 hours of fasting can reset the immune system in their mice test subjects. The process generates blood cells in the body and promotes immunity. Fasting from 3 to 5 days is the optimal time frame for autophagy and prevents the onset of relapse among people. Although this type of fasting is not needed and ill-advised for some, it can do wonders for your body in terms of longevity, health, and immunity once you have accomplished this.

## 8. Alternate-Day Fasting

Alternate-day fasting is also known as the 5:2 diet as it allows consumption of approximately 500 calories on days when you can merely eat small portions of food during the eating window. By restricting your caloric intake, however, it makes the physiological effects of fasting more difficult to kick in. Plus, there's a greater tendency for you to miscalculate the number of calories taken during the day. Furthermore, there's a greater risk of losing self-discipline or trying to binge-eat.

## 9. Fasting Mimicking Diet

The ninth type of intermittent fasting is the fasting mimicking diet in which a person can eat 800 to 1000 calories a day for 2-5 days in a month. After that, you can return to a normal eating schedule starting from day 6. This type of intermittent fasting is known to reduce blood pressure, lower insulin level, and suppress IGF-1, which are all related to a person's longevity. When you follow this method, you're only allowed to eat foods with low protein, moderate carbs, and fats, such as mushroom soup, olives, nut bars, kale, and others. The idea is to make your caloric intake as low as possible and to avoid autophagy. But then again, there are downsides of doing this technique just like with alternate-day fasting.

## 10. Protein-Sparing Modified Diet

Protein-sparing modified diet is one of the least common forms of intermittent fasting. The method requires you to eat food with high protein content but low carbohydrates and fats. This is essential for bodybuilders who only want to lose weight and burn fat without the risk of autophagy. It also helps maintain leans muscles and make sure that you do not take more protein than what your body can take.

## 11. Fat Fasting

This form of intermittent fasting is known to be "fat fasting." Considering you have heard about the ketogenic diet, you should know that the effects of fasting and the keto diet are the same. It is only the methods that differ. Both of these facilitate the metabolic state of ketosis or the process of burning down fats when the liver no longer has glucose to spare for the body. This enables a person to acquire energy for the whole day. If you think that eating loads of fat will get your body out of ketosis, you are wrong. It might increase the amount of fat in your body, but it does not necessarily mean that the metabolic state will end.

## 12. Bone Broth Fasting

This is a method for intermittent fasting that allows you to extend fasting for a longer period of time. Bone broth contains amino acids that inhibit autophagy in the body. For fat loss, you will not want to consume large amounts of calories because it strips down the essence of losing weight. One cup of bone broth will suffice to give you the energy that you need to complete your daily activities. Furthermore, the electrolytes and minerals from bone broth are essential for preventing brain fog, lethargy, and muscle cramps.

## 13. Dry-Fasting

Dry-fasting is a form of intermittent fasting that prevents the intake of any form of liquid. This might be one of the most difficult types of fasting since most people cannot live without rehydration from time to time. Others, however, can live without solid food for days at a time with the assistance of water, juice, coffee, tea, and other beverages. However, there are only a few who can survive days without rehydrating their body. There is a theory that states that dry-fasting is equal to three days of water fasting. The concept is that when the body is deprived of any liquid, the body will start to reproduce its own by converting triglycerides from the adipose tissues or fats into metabolic water. Triglycerides are the main constituent of body fat in humans and animals.

Did you know that dry-fasting is a method of healing in some religious beliefs? This method includes restricted fasting for a time frame of 12 to 16 hours for maximum effects.

## 14. Juice Fasting

For a long time, I have never thought that juice fasting is a thing, but it really works! This method refers to using vegetables and fruits that ensure the intake of a significant amount of carbohydrates and fructose, which is essential in providing energy to the body. The idea of green and power smoothies can be associated with this kind of intermittent fasting. Researchers have found that someone can lose a significant amount of weight using juice fasting while promoting the buildup of lean muscle mass.

## 15. Time-Restricted Feeding

The last form of intermittent fasting is known as time-restricted feeding. This technique has originated from the popularization of circadian rhythms and chronobiology, which aims to restrict a person's daily food intake. According to further experiments, this type reduces the onset of metabolic disorders among humans and animals. On a more specific note, the mice that had been fed for eight hours did not get obese or develop any chronic disease as compared to those that were fed with the same number of calories without time restrictions. Simply put, when you aim to eat 1000 calories per day, avoid eating it in one sitting when you can diversify its intake in the span of 8 hours per day. Not only will this help you build a good sense of self-discipline but it will also boost your metabolism.

# CHAPTER 3:

## THE 30-DAY CHALLENGE

In the previous chapters, we have discussed the importance of fasting to people. Whether it is about weight loss, longevity or even prevention of several illnesses such as cardiovascular diseases, respiratory diseases, diabetes, and many more. When I first heard the idea of fasting, I honestly felt a bit skeptic about it. There were thoughts running within my mind saying that I might acquire ulcer from this or that I might develop more illnesses because the practice could crash my immune system. When I did some research, though, I was surprised to find out that the effects of fasting were quite the opposite.

The reason why I want to include a 30-day challenge for fasting is that it has really worked for me, given the right method of intermittent fasting. During the month of December 2018, it was inevitable to join several parties in a row. There was drinking and so much eating, especially during Christmas and New Year. It was difficult for me to abstain because I grew up in a family where social gatherings are very important. I couldn't simply decline their offer to eat because it would be rude. However, I engaged in voracious eating and drinking not because I couldn't say no but because I liked it. And I thought, "You only live once." That year was a rough one for me because I was diagnosed with nephritis or the inflammation of the nephrons in the kidney. Before that, I was diagnosed with angina and gastroesophageal reflux disorder. My doctor recommended having small amounts of food every now and then, especially when I felt like my stomach was building up too much acid. Eating and drinking excessively were detrimental, too. I was not allowed to consume food with salt or vinegar since they irritate the kidneys. This frustrated me during that holiday season, but I decided to do it because I was hard-headed. The downside was that everything got worse after the New Year when I felt every effect of the unhealthy lifestyle I emancipated last December. I grew stout and noticed a significant decline in my immune system. My parents thought that I was getting healthier. In fact, however, my situation got worse. So, I decided to fast.

Food abstinence was the most difficult challenge for me because I was hungry all the time. To gain a little bit of self-control, therefore, I would distract myself every now and then. After days of research, I found out that there were other methods of fasting. Nevertheless, in my case, intermittent fasting worked the best to reduce weight and regain my healthy body. It was difficult to assess which specific tactic to use in fasting. But then, I realized that I had been doing it subconsciously even without scheduling or setting up alarms. After all, I was getting sick. My loss of appetite made me believe the concept of Hippocrates about food abstinence when a person was ill. From this, I decided to continue this 16/8 method for a whole month. Of course, in the beginning, I couldn't believe that it was possible. I thought that sooner or later, I would be tempted to eat a lot of food again. But as I ventured and persevered daily, I realized that I slowly developed control over my urges. I felt a sense of satiation, too, so I did not feel too hungry anymore unless my body would signal that it's time to eat.

After a month, I noticed a workable improvement in my health. I lost a couple of pounds, and I no longer felt pain on my lower back, which indicated kidney problems. At first, I thought that my GERD would worsen because of fasting. It turned out that, with the help of various healthy beverages, I was able to overcome this illness as well. Angina and heartburn did not bother me either. Thus, I did not intend to stop even when my 30-day challenge was already over.

Now, it is time for you to enjoy the same benefits that I do now by starting your own 30-day challenge. First and foremost, you need to assess the kind of method that you will be employing. You may refer to the types of intermittent fasting in the previous chapter if you are unsure of what to choose and figure out what is best for you. Furthermore, you should consider several factors.

## 1. Your Daily Schedule

Assess the time frame when you are free to eat. Base your intermittent fasting schedule to your work, school, and other daily activities. This way, your body will be able to adjust quickly with the changes. And if it is time to break your fast, you can maintain a healthy eat-fast period.

## 2. Your Daily Routine

What are the tasks that you need to complete every day? The answer defines the time when you should eat. For example, you do heavy work in the morning, so it is best to have your meals as early as 6 A.M. before fasting after that. However, if you are working late at night, it is advisable to eat at around 6 to 7 P.M. so that you'll have energy to get through your activities.

3. Your Body Rhythm

Assess yourself and determine the hours when you feel hungriest. From this, you can schedule your eating periods on time and fast during the remaining hours of the day. Say, if you're used to skipping breakfast, you can start fasting at around 10 A.M. or lunchtime. In that way, you can successfully perform a full fast for the rest of the day or until your next eating period.

So, what should you expect when you start your 30-day challenge? Well, I am sure that we all experience the side effects of fasting on different notes. More often than not, though, the first week is the most challenging because this is when your body starts to adapt to the changes brought by food abstinence. The side effects may include headaches, bowel movements, cravings, and thirst, among others. Much like any other method, you will experience some drawbacks in the beginning. However, this shouldn't be something to be alarmed about. When you start noticing such effects, it is best to stay hydrated during most of the fasting hours. Once you go to work or school, you can bring water or green smoothies with you. This will help you develop a faster metabolism and speed up the process of autophagy.

During the second week, you may experience headaches as your body tries to accommodate your new diet. There's a greater need to satiate your thirst as well; that's why you need to have a lot of water. You can incorporate low-carb drinks such as grapefruit juice, cranberry juice, and other forms of healthy beverages. During the third week, you may feel the preliminary effects of intermittent fasting. You will start to lose weight and notice that you no longer crave for food as much as you have before fasting. You can feel a significant increase in your metabolism and mental sharpness. In the fourth week, your body will have accommodated the process and crave for intermittent fasting more. You will soon enjoy the effects of fasting such as alertness, better skin and hair health, enhanced immune system and metabolism, and, of course, a remarkable weight loss.

# CHAPTER 4:
# QUICK START GUIDE


Now that you know what to look after while fasting intermittently, it is time to learn a quick guideline regarding the method. We have discussed in the previous chapter the several factors that you need to understand in order to schedule your new routine. In this chapter, we will be digging deeper into the different techniques to make intermittent fasting more convenient for you.

We all have different kinds of routines every day. As a worker, student, mother, or a pioneer, we always have to deal with a plethora of activities. Sometimes, no matter how much we try so much to engage in intermittent fasting, our schedule does not permit us to do so. Hence, it is very important to assess our time and foster self-management.

You read it right! You need self-management to make a successful intermittent fasting schedule. First and foremost, let us dig more into the term 'self-management.' In all honesty, I do not like to use the word "time-management" that often. Because, somehow, I believe that people cannot really manage time. There are 24 hours in a day, seven days in a week, and 365 and ¼ days in a year, and I do not think that you are equipped with the power to change it or at least slow it down. In truth, none of us can do that. This is merely a misconception from our end. The reality is that it is not the time that we manage; instead, it is ourselves and how we present ourselves to the circumstances of the restricted time, which allows us to manage our activities and finish things on time.

In this chapter, I will be discussing the importance of self-management when you are trying to do intermittent fasting successfully, as well as how you can manage yourself to be effective in your weight-loss journey. Self-management is known to be a vital factor when it comes to self-improvement and self-mastery. It empowers discovery, innovation, resourcefulness, and success in everything that you do. This term refers to how an individual behaves in whatever activity that he or she has to do. Self-management is very much associated with commitment, planning, decisiveness, productivity, and organization, all of which are essential to intermittent fasting. A person needs to learn how to manage himself or herself while emancipating a hint of motivation to support his or her ideas in the midst of any challenge. Self-management is also a manner of nurturing your personal network. When you can practice self-management, you may feel more inclined to understand your actions a little deeper. You may also become more willing than ever to accept and own up to your mistakes. Not to mention, you will be able to help people in the middle of any adversity, share your success to others, and pull them up for their own self-improvement.

It is easy to say that you have commitment and ability to manage yourself. However, it is way easier said than done. Most people in this world who have achieved success in their goals and dreams are reported to have a huge amount of self-management in their system. To develop this value, you need to apply simple steps in your daily living.

## 1. Stay Positive

"Think positive" - that's what many individuals always say. If I earn a penny every time I hear this short saying, I may already be living in a mansion now. Despite that observe and look at the people who genuinely embody positivity in their lives. These two words are not challenging to pronounce, but it is difficult to apply when push comes to shove, and the circumstances become too tough to handle. Why do you think this quote came to life in the first place? It is to provide a motivation to folks no matter how hard their trials may be.

It is important to stay positive even when you have problems, and so you need to feel more inclined to think critically, decide, and solve problems efficiently. Maintaining a positive mind can reduce your anxiety, frustration, and stress, which are huge factors that brings down a person. Positivity prevents you from breaking down and giving up. It puts your issues in a new light, giving you hope that it is merely temporary. While you are trying to pull off a successful intermittent fasting schedule, it is inevitable to experience several forms of mishaps and shortcomings. However, when you think positively about your routine, you will see how easily these circumstances can be solved.

## 2. Learn to Manage Stress

There are people out there who deal with emotional breakdown in the midst of extreme stress. That's why you should learn how to manage yourself even when you are facing worries and anxiety. When people think about stress, they often see it negatively. In fact, there is a positive outcome of being stressed: it pushes a person to move forward and get things done. That is, if people know how to manage their minds during stressful moments. But when stress is present, and they think about it with pure negativity, they have a greater tendency to break down and stop trying. Stress and fasting do not add up peacefully in our system. When we are stressed, it is our first instinct to compensate for these feelings with sugary foods, which is something that we cannot do during our fasting hours. This might leave us hangry (or angry because of hunger). This is the reason why we need to learn how to manage these emotions. Here are a few hacks to manage yourself during stressful times.

### Avoid Caffeine

Caffeine is known to increase the amount of cortisol in the body, which is responsible for increasing your stress levels. If you are a coffee person, it is recommended to shift your beverage preference to tea and juice from time to time, especially when you do not feel okay.

### Stay Physically Active

Exercising is a good way to reduce your stress levels because it helps boost the endorphins or "feel-good" hormone in the body.

### Learn to Distract Yourself

When you are feeling stressed, do not make matters worse by engaging in strenuous work. You know yourself too well. You have an idea when you are getting stressed out. Thus, you should distract yourself with other activities that can alleviate the tension in your body. Learn to rest when you get a break time; go out and enjoy the fresh air every now and then.

## Acknowledge Your Emotions

There are instances when we fail to acknowledge our emotions, primarily when we feel stressed or frustrated. Neglecting or repressing your feelings and thoughts, however, can worsen your situation. The main reason why people experience burnout is that the cramped-up emotions are buried within their hearts. It only takes one emotional trigger to unleash all of them at once, and it can take a toll on your psychological and social well-being. So, whenever you feel stressed, let it out immediately. Never invalidate your feelings just because it seems negative. Embrace it and allow it to be a part of you. This way, you will understand yourself more and be able to live better and let things go easier.

## Talk to People

One of the most important ways to destress is to talk to people about random things. You can open up to them regarding your darkest secrets if you want. Nevertheless, by surrounding yourself with happy people, you get injected with the happy serum as well. You start to see things differently and feel happy about yourself.

## Be Responsible for Your Actions

Another common mistake is blaming other people and events for their mistakes and shortcomings. When you aim to become efficient at managing yourself, you need to start to own up to your mistakes and learn from them instead of pointing your finger to every other person on the planet except for yourself. Think of it this way: would you rather remain stagnant by pointing fingers at each other or stay productive and search for a solution?

### *Avoid Procrastinating*

Procrastination is like a black hole that dulls the mind and lessens the motivation of a person. It is one of the most dangerous pits that no one can normally rise from. Whenever you feel the need to stay lazy, get up and do something about it. Never let your dull emotions cloud your rationality, especially if you have a goal to achieve. This is also a common problem among people who are trying to lose weight. Instead of going to the gym or doing home workouts, they choose to be a couch potato. Procrastination tells the mind that a certain activity is "so difficult" even when it is manageable. Watch out for this type of issue! It can destroy all of your routines, including intermittent fasting.

### *Do Not Wait for Monday*

Start now! Do not wait for the right moment to start. If you want to do something, do it already. How sure are you that you will be as motivated on Monday? Do not entertain the "what-if" questions in your head because they will cause you to fail. Instead, use your current drive to make the first step.

# HOW TO SCHEDULE YOUR FASTING

## 1. Stay Focused on Your Goals

It helps to have a daily reminder of your goals and objectives every now and then. Remember when I told you to keep a journal? It is best to have it with you all the time to have a physical remembrance of the schedule that you should follow for intermittent fasting. As much as possible, avoid any activity that can derail you from doing the routine. Realize its temporariness so that you can withstand any challenge that life may throw at you.

## 2. Use a Calendar

Utilize the calendar feature on your phone or computer. You can even acquire a hard copy of the calendar where you can write your upcoming events and organize your agendas beforehand. Having one for intermittent fasting can help you track your progress during a 30-day challenge as well. For example, mark the days green when you have successfully employed intermittent fasting. At the same time, indicate what you felt, what you ate, and what you plan to do the next day. You can also have a customized calendar where you can write motivational quotes and boost your energy. When you think you have failed for the day, mark your calendar orange or red and mention the challenges that you have faced. However, instead of feeling guilty, use these shortcomings as a mode of learning for future reference. Indicate the solutions that you can try, to be specific, when dire situations come up so that you will not repeat the same mistakes again.

## 3. Use an Alarm

It is best to set your alarm 10 to 15 minutes before breaking your fast. This is to ready yourself for the food that you are about to eat. It helps you to set your mindset and gain control over the next activities. Another advantage of keeping an alarm is that when your body has finally accustomed to the specific time to eat and fast, it can become your own alarm clock. It will synchronize itself and allow you to stick to an effective schedule of eating and fasting. This way, you no longer have to set an alarm, and your body will always be alert.

## 4. Schedule Fast Breaks

Schedule your fast breaks accordingly. Whether you are a worker or a student, after all, there is a specific time when you can get some lunch or rest from your activities within the day. To make fasting a lot easier to adopt, you can set your breaks during this time to avoid any hindrances in your daily activities.

## 5. Plan Ahead of Time

Most people disregard the importance of planning ahead of time. In fact, this method will allow you to schedule your tasks more successfully. It is best to plan things one day before it happens. For example, for my fasting routine for tomorrow, I will eat avocado at 10 A.M. as a snack. I might be able to grab some on the way to work as well. When you set things one or two days before it happens, it allows your mind to settle with the idea of doing such an activity. So, when the time comes, you are less likely to procrastinate because your mind is already set to do it.

## 6. Don't Waste Time

One of the main reasons why people have constricted time is their inability to ward off procrastination. The most dangerous word to think about when scheduling and trying to do self-management is 'later' since it comes with no sense of definiteness. It can take hours or days before a person can actually accomplish something if you always use this word. When you have the chance to do something at once, maximize your time to do so to be able to do more things in the future.

# CHAPTER 5:
# DOS AND DON'TS WHILE
# FASTING INTERMITTENTLY

Weight loss is something that you may think about if you feel too bad about the size of your body. Hence, you might start looking for different diets to try. According to the World Health Organization (WHO) in 2016, there were more than 1.9 billion people across the globe who were overweight. More than 650 million individuals, on the other hand, were obese, and this case had tripled in number since 1975. With a high number of people dealing with obesity, there are weight-loss programs that have been done in hopes of reducing this count. These plans have been developed to help someone achieve their ideal physique.

As we have discussed in the earlier chapters, some people use intermittent fasting for detoxification, treatment of several medical conditions, weight loss, and conformation to certain religious practices. For instance, the Muslims fast during Ramadan. Intermittent fasting is a diet regimen that involves alternating cycles of fasting and eating. In simpler terms, you make a mindful decision to skip meals on purpose when you follow this method. Generally, intermittent fasting means that an individual consumes calories during a specific time of the day and prefers not to eat an ample amount of food for a longer period. Aside from weight loss, studies also show that this can help improve your metabolic health and protect you against diseases. However, in order to maximize these benefits, you must be able to carry out intermittent fasting efficiently. There are some instances when people complain about the lack of effectiveness of the method. The reason is that that they are unable to execute the proper procedure of intermittent fasting. For this chapter, therefore, it seems important to discuss the dos and don'ts of intermittent fasting to help you get better results. There are other methods to be followed as well in order to execute such practice without sacrificing your health. As what many practitioners say, fasting is good as long as you know how to discipline yourself, when it should be done, and how to avoid abusing it.

# THE DOS OF INTERMITTENT FASTING

## *Make A Plan*

Intermittent fasting comes with different options, such as 24-hour fasting, skipping meals for 16 hours or having one meal per day. It is best to know which mealtime planning is best for you and what method suits your body well. Other people talk with their doctor before deciding what technique what makes the most sense, and that's something that you should do as well.

## *Make Sure You Are Fit to Fast*

Make sure that you are fit to fast to avoid sacrificing your health for this method. You should not even thinking of fasting if you are pregnant, lactating, diabetics, or below the age of 18. Of course, it is not recommendable to individuals with underlying medical problems or those who are taking prescription drugs to evade erratic reactions in the body.

## *Prepare Your Mind and Body*

Guarantee that you are in good condition and have a well-rested mind and body before proceeding with the technique. It is important to be able to focus on your goal, your reason for fasting. Preparing your body and mind can allow you to sustain the time of fasting and not feel weak easily.

## Drink Lots of Water

It is important to stay hydrated while fasting as well. Proper hydration can help restrain you from feeling hungry. Water fasting, to be specific, helps promote autophagy, a process wherein the body breaks down and recycles old parts of the cells that may potentially be dangerous. Keeping yourself hydrated can keep you going and prevent you from dealing with an empty stomach all the time.

## Listen to Your Body

While intermittent fasting comes with many benefits, it is still important to listen to what your body is feeling. Getting dizzy or weak while fasting can affect your ability to be productive and complete your tasks. You should only fast you feel healthy so that the food restrictions will not stress you out or make you feel fatigued and irritated.

## Be Patient

Sometimes, people start fasting and think about how badly they want to lose body fats. With this mindset, they tend to avoid eating for a day or at any time of the day and keep on skipping meals. When these folks can no longer stand their hunger, they try to restrict their caloric intake severely. Although you can be strict or mindful of your diet, you should also refrain from depriving yourself of food when you are allowed to eat. Keep in mind that there are always healthy options to choose from after your fasting time is over.

## Eat Enough Protein

Registered dietitian Molly Devine said that most people should be able to consume adequate protein amounts during an eight-hour feeding window. When fasting, excellent sources of protein like beef, chicken and fish can be had for two meals to obtain enough protein for the body and prevent muscle wasting. It is important to aim for at least 4 to 6 ounces of protein daily. Some studies show that consuming around 30% of protein can significantly lessen your appetite. Therefore, eating some meat and other protein sources on fasting days can offset some of its side effects.

## Eat Plenty of Whole Foods on Non-Fasting Days

Maintaining a healthy lifestyle on non-fasting days is recommended. It is necessary to eat plenty of whole foods like meat, fish, eggs, vegetables, and fruits when you are not fasting because healthy diets based on them are linked to a wide range of health benefits, including a reduced risk of cancer, heart disease, and other chronic illnesses. The author of *The Protein-Packed Breakfast Club*, Lauren Harris-Pincus, said that anyone attempting to lose weight should focus on nutrient-dense foods, such as fruits, veggies, whole grains, nuts, beans, seeds, dairy, and lean proteins. Eating these kinds of foods on non-fasting days will keep you on track.

## Consider Taking Supplements

Taking supplements is advised if you fast regularly since there are essential nutrients that you may miss out when you depend on the foods that you consume. Eating fewer calories regularly can make it harder for you to meet your nutritional needs, you see. Therefore, it is necessary to supplement your diet with calcium, iron or any multivitamin to prevent mineral deficiencies.

## Stay Physically Active

Doing exercise while intermittent fasting basically forces the body to shed fat, considering the latter process is controlled by the sympathetic nervous system (SNS), which gets activated by exercise and lack of food. A certain study found that fasting before aerobic training leads to both body weight and fat reduction. Eating before a workout, on the other hand, merely decreases your body weight. The combination of fasting and exercising maximizes the impact of cellular factors and catalysts (cyclic AMP and AMP Kinases), which force the breakdown of fat and glycogen for energy.

# THE DON'TS OF INTERMITTENT FASTING

While there are positive things to keep in mind while fasting intermittently, there are also ideas that you should avoid no matter what.

## *Fasting If You Have Health Conditions*

It is important to consider a healthy condition when doing fasting. According to Anne Brock, who specializes in weight loss and diabetic education, those people with type 1 and 2 diabetes, children, teens, and pregnant or nursing women should avoid intermittent fasting. It is necessary to follow such a rule because doing so with an unhealthy body might lead to severe consequences. Instead of helping, this might worsen your health.

## *Don't Overindulge the Night Before*

Avoid overindulging in a fatty meal such as fries or burgers before starting a fast. Instead, slow-burning nutrients are recommended to be supplemented to the body. Anne Brock has also said that it is advisable to get some carbohydrates, protein, and unsaturated fats in order to ensure that you are getting nutrient-dense foods rather than varieties that are rich in trans fats.

## *Don't Work Out Too Hard*

Performing any high-intensity workouts during a fast should be avoided; instead, you should only do light to moderate exercises. One study states eating combining low-intensity workouts with 20% to 25% of the participants' regular calories for two days per week has resulted in superior weight loss compared to fasting or exercising alone. Nevertheless, it is important to make sure that you are getting 25% of the required calories daily so that your muscle mass will not deplete." It is quite difficult to expend energy that you do not regain through eating; that's why you have look for a suitable workout routine that matches your intermittent fasting to maximize the results.

## *Don't Stress Yourself Out*

Your level of stress can increase while fasting because some hormones might be triggered when you think too much about getting fast results. Stress boosts your cortisol level, a certain hormone that stores fat and breaks down muscle. It will be beneficial to practice de-stressing techniques such as yoga, deep breathing or meditation. Make sure that it is not too strenuous if you decide to calm down by doing an exercise, too. After all, to be able to function throughout the day, you need to reserve your energy.

While intermittent fasting has been globally popularized as a method to lose weight and prepare a healthy meal plan, there are still factors to consider before doing it. Following the dos and don'ts above can make you feel more confident about fasting and making it more effective.

# CHAPTER 6:

# MOTHERS' GUIDE TO INTERMITTENT FASTING

Gaining weight while you are pregnant is what most expectant mothers worry about. Although some moms tend to shrug off the idea of gaining wait, there are still women who feel too conscious about their physique and want to bring back their pre-pregnancy body immediately. Some go on exercise, while others merely do not have time to do so. Most mothers put the needs of their children first, so they might not be able to take care of themselves like they used to before having kids.

Researchers conducted a study on nearly 30,000 women who had given birth between one and four times and found out that most of them never got their pre-pregnancy body weight back after giving birth. Some studies reveal that moms find it difficult to lose weight after the delivery even with breastfeeding; thus, they continue to gain weight. Just two weeks after the birth of their children, 63% of all women wish to return to their pre-pregnancy size and shape. Not every mother knows about the risks of doing so, however. There are issues recorded about new moms who have developed low thyroid function during and after pregnancy, as well as sleeplessness and stress, and they have all contributed to postpartum weight gain.

An associate professor from the University of Michigan named Olga Yakusheva conducted a research about women gaining weight, too. She realized that the reason why many mothers have higher rates of weight gain is that there was a change in their lifestyle. Furthermore, the study showed that that typical age-related weight gain for women is about 1.94 pounds a year, while those females with toddlers garnered almost a full pound annually.

Despite the fact that a lot of mothers are contented with their current physique, some may still prefer to find ways to lose weight. In this case, diet may be the first choice. The problem is that the current weight-loss trend that has become popular over the years is intermittent fasting, a method that requires you to go in and out of fasting mode depending on the type that you decide to take on. Question is, is it advisable for you?

There are women who experience missed periods, metabolic disturbances, and even early onset of menopause when doing intermittent fasting. However, this fasting technique can work for some ladies, especially mothers. The important thing to really consider is how it should be done. There are certain ways to do it, so you have a few options in your hands. Because your children will always be your top priority, and you should attend to their needs, there are certain tips to be followed to help you schedule your fast more conveniently.

1. Choose the right fasting hours

As a mom, household chores can undoubtedly keep you busy. For working women, your workload can add to your priorities. Nevertheless, you can still aim to lose weight by choosing the right fasting hours. You should define your hunger patterns and up to what extent you can continue fasting. Remember that you do not have to deprive yourself of food and drinks if you think that you cannot handle it. Any time of the day that works best for you is recommended. Figuring out the right fasting hours for yourself will set you up for success.

2. Determine the best fasting method

There are different fasting methods to choose from. Since mothers mostly do a lot of chores at home or office, you should merely focus on finding the right fasting technique. One popular practice is the 16/8 method wherein you need to fast for 16 hours each day and restrict your daily "eating window" to 8 hours. Another technique is the 5:2 diet wherein you have to consume 500 to 600 calories for 2 days per week and eat normally in the next 5 days. The eat-stop-eat method can also be done, although it entails that you have to do a 24-hour fast once or twice a week. Alternate-day fasting is a different technique that allows you to fast every other day, while the warrior diet lets you fast during the day and eat a huge meal at night. Spontaneous meal skipping, on the other hand, means that you can avoid eating whenever it feels convenient to you. It is not necessary to follow a structured intermittent fasting plan, but you have to consider the best method that you can handle. After, such a factor might affect your weight-loss goals, as well as your duties as a wife, mother or employee.

3. Make healthy food choices

Fasting works best when healthy food choices are considered. Though you need to abstain from eating or drinking up to a certain period depending on the fasting method chosen, you should opt for healthy options when you can do either. The craving for fast food or comfort food can really take over and increase the difficulty of making such choices. Some healthy foods to consider while fasting are low-carb vegetables, nuts and seeds, smoothies, and fruits like berries and avocados. Mothers, in particular, must find the balance that is the best for them to lose the post-baby weight. If cutting carbs and adding more protein and fats to their diet can boost their energy level and fend off cravings, they should do that. By sticking to healthy food while fasting, it may allow you to see the results faster than ever.

## 4. Stay hydrated

Drinking lots of water is essential when you follow the intermittent fasting technique. As a mom, you should always stay hydrated to be able to function throughout the day. Water can promote a better flow of blood, cognition, and muscle and joint support during the regimen. Avoid consuming diet drinks, though, because they merely contain artificial sweeteners. Some studies have shown a potential links between artificial sweeteners, increased appetite, and over-consumption, and they wreak havoc on your insulin levels and set back the entire purpose of fasting.

## 5. Take multivitamins

Since most mothers have a lot of duties to deal with, be it at home or in the office, starving themselves might not be helpful because they risk having vitamin deficiency. A daily intake of multivitamins might be the key to staying healthy while fasting intermittently. A practical advice to some women, especially those who are still breastfeeding, is to continue taking the vitamins that your doctor recommends.

## 6. Get more sleep

It might be difficult for mothers with a newborn baby to get more sleep, but it is essential if you are eyeing to follow a weight-loss plan and get better results. If you cannot stay inactive for longer hours, at least try to get a better quality of rest. The reason is that sleep is interconnected with our hunger pattern. Doing intermittent fasting can make the brain more active, which leads to the difficulty of falling asleep. Thus, a sleep routine must be set. Your body might adjust to the new plan, so you will have time to self-contemplate and detoxify your body. The more rejuvenated you feel, the clearer your thinking pattern is and the deeper you should be able to sleep. To loosen up your muscles and help the detoxification process, you can get a massage before your bedtime. Alternatively, you may try drinking green tea or chamomile tea to calm your nerves at night.

## 7. Exercise

According to Chelsea Amengual, the manager of Fitness Programming & Nutrition at Virtual Health Partners at the time of writing this guide, it is possible that your body will start to break down muscle to use protein for fuel while exercising in a fasted state. Plus, you are more susceptible to hitting the wall at this moment, which means that you will have less energy to work out as hard or perform as well as you have done before. However, as you adjust to the new eating pattern, it is important to be reminded that your training must not be overdone. While exercising regularly, you should increase its intensity gradually so as not to shock the body. Some experts also recommend exercising immediately before breaking the fast to reap the greatest metabolic benefits. Mothers have certain exercise options to consider, too, such as walking, swimming, and yoga. You are free to try any or all of them to see what gives the most ideal results.

While some people only think about intermittent fasting as an essential weight-loss tool, it comes with other benefits, such as providing healthy metabolism, activating the "cleanup mode," improving cognitive skills and memory function, enhancing immunity, lowering inflammation, and boosting longevity genes. It is difficult to guarantee how well or badly the method will work for you. If you decide to give intermittent fasting a try, you must make sure to listen to your body's feedback because easing into this fasting technique by skipping a meal or two every day might lead to initial symptoms of hunger and discomfort. If the system refuses to respond positively and causes you to feel uncomfortably, it is better to accept it and move on to other programs. In the end, your well-being should be one of your top priorities. Mothers wanting to lose weight through fasting, in particular, should be more mindful of their body and not abuse it since the kids need them. This idea is especially true for moms with newborn babies. You ought to be physically, mentally, and emotionally healthy while fasting to garner better results and avoid sacrificing yourself.

# CHAPTER 7:

# WHAT TO EAT WHILE DOING

# INTERMITTENT FASTING

Every woman on a diet is supposed to plan what meals to eat for a day ahead of time. However, the procedure cannot be the same if we start talking about intermittent fasting. For one, not everyone may be familiar of the technique, even though it merely involves abstaining from consuming foods and drinks for a certain period of time. Not only has it been practiced recently but our ancestors have tried fasting back then as well. While most people in the olden times prefer fasting for religious purposes, it is on this era that the has become a trend for health and fitness reasons. Losing weight is something that someone who feels heavier than usually will most likely aim to do with the help of some dietary actions, including fasting. So, you can tell that intermittent fasting is not merely a fad.

Now, despite choosing not to eat or drink while fasting, it does not necessarily mean that you no longer have a chance to consume anything throughout this period. Of course, you can still do it; otherwise, you will starve yourself and deprive your body of nutrients that come from healthy foods. Although we are on a dietary plan, we should know what varieties to eat and avoid. The main question here is: are you willing to drop the unhealthy foods and drinks you used to love in the name of fasting? Are you willing to give up burgers and fries and ice cream for quite some time? For people who do not like vegetables, this might be a rough patch for you. Giving up the things that make you happy can be quite a pain - that is true. However, with the right motivation, I believe you can survive the ordeal, especially if you want to shed extra pounds.

What should you eat while you are doing the intermittent fasting, you may ask? There are certain food varieties that have been found to be ideal for consumption when you follow this method. These foods and beverages are listed as follows:

### *Water*

The most common advice for a person who is fasting intermittently is to drink lots of water to stay hydrated. Promoting hydration helps our body to continue functioning throughout the day. As we go through a period of abstaining from food from 12 to 16 hours, you have no choice but to use up glycogen, the sugar stored in the liver, for energy. As this energy gets burned, the amount of electrolytes and fluids in the body will decrease significantly. We are always told to drink at least 8 glasses of water per day to prevent dehydration and promote a better flow of blood, cognition, and muscle and joint support while doing intermittent fasting. Water is always the best choice to drink all day long. If you are not a fan of water, a lemon can be added as flavor to your water, as well as cucumber or orange slices. However, do not use any artificially-sweetened water enhancers such as Crystal Light because this will wreak havoc on your insulin levels and may cause you to gain weight in the process.

## Coffee

This beverage is known to be a calorie-free drink. It is suitable to get your blood flowing in the morning, and it is important to kick-start your day. While your stomach might get acidic when you drink coffee on an empty stomach, you can use the beverage as an alternative for soft drinks, which are filled with sugar. Did you know that black coffee can enhance the detoxification benefits of intermittent fasting? It can also improve your body's insulin sensitivity in the long run. Remember that you can drink coffee, provided that you do not mix cream, milk or sweeteners with it.

## Minimally-Processed Foods

Carbohydrates can trigger someone on a diet, in the sense that whenever they hear this word, they most likely give an eerie reaction. Of course, too many carbs can genuinely have a negative impact on our body, especially when our goal is to lose weight. While fasting, it is essential to think strategically on how to get the adequate calories that you need without feeling overly full. Though it is advised to minimize the consumption of processed foods, there can be a time and place for such items like crackers, whole-grain bread, and bagels. These types of foods are more likely to be quickly digested; thus, they are recommendable as fast and easy fuel sources of our body. Other foods to consider can be bagged spinach, sliced vegetables, and roasted nuts, and they can be pre-prepped for convenience. These minimally processed foods can also help if you intend to exercise while fasting intermittently even when you are on the road.

## Tea

Known as a health elixir in many ancient cultures, tea has been a powerhouse enhancer, especially for a intermittent fasting lifestyle. If your fast calls for no energy-source intake, which means avoid sugar, milk or cream on any of your beverages, tea is the next best thing to turn to. According to a 2018 study, unsweetened herbal teas have been used widely due to their hydrating effect. There are different types of tea to try during a fast, namely green, black, oolong and herbal. However, research has proven that green tea helps to suppress appetite and enhance weight loss. In general, tea can boost the effectiveness of intermittent fasting by promoting gut health, probiotic balance, and cellular detoxification.

## Apple Cider Vinegar

Another great drink for fasting is apple cider vinegar, which has anti-bacterial and anti-inflammatory compounds that can combat various health issues. Although this product is acidic, it helps in balancing the body's pH levels. No calories are found in apple cider vinegar, but this has minerals like potassium, magnesium, and iron. This can also lower blood sugar level, improve digestion, eliminate bad bacteria, and stave off hunger.

## Potatoes

Like bread, the body can digest white potatoes with minimal effort. When paired with a protein source, it becomes a perfect post-workout snack to refuel your hungry muscles and energy. Potatoes can be a good source of many vitamins and minerals, such as potassium and vitamin C, especially if you cook them with skin. This is also high in the water content when fresh, although a potato mainly composes of carbs and contains moderate amounts of protein and fiber (but almost no fat). Furthermore, another benefit of making potatoes a part of intermittent fasting is that once cooled, potatoes can form a resistant starch primer that can fuel the good bacteria in your gut.

## Soybeans

Soybeans contain a number of health benefits that come from the nutrients, vitamins, and organic compounds, including a significant amount of dietary fiber and protein. Common to Asian diets, soybeans play an important role in cuisines as they have been consumed even thousands of years ago. According to the USDA National Nutrient Database, soybeans comprise of vitamin K, riboflavin, folate, vitamin B6, thiamin, and vitamin C. Moreover, they are also a good source of organic compounds and antioxidants, which further help in boosting your well-being. Soybeans mainly grow in Asia and South and North America. In addition to that, there is one active compound found in soybeans, a.k.a. the isoflavones, which has been demonstrated to inhibit UVB-induced cell damage and promote anti-aging.

## Nuts and Seeds

While fasting, another source of energy can be nuts and seeds. They may include Macadamia nuts, flaxseed, Brazil nuts, chia seeds, walnuts, pecans, hemp seeds, hazelnuts, sesame seeds, pumpkin seeds, and almonds. Nuts and seeds are excellent sources for protein, and they are easy on the digestive tract. However, do not eat more than a handful of nuts and seeds at a time. The proper discipline of eating some sources of energy on fasting is still best to keep in mind.

## Multivitamins

The reason why a lot of individuals prefer to do intermittent fasting to lose weight is that the approach requires less time to eat. However, one should know how to follow this method properly. For one, starving yourself by choice may not be have a good effect to your body. While we keep disregarding our source of energy by skipping meals, there might be a risk of vitamin deficiency while in a caloric deficit. Nevertheless, this does not mean that you have to take as many supplements as you can afford. It is merely advisable to take multivitamins at some point because your body might not function well if you fast too much. Though a multivitamin is not necessary with a balanced diet that consists of plenty of fruits and vegetables, life can get hectic, and a supplement can help fill the gaps.

## Seafood

This food group is rich in B vitamins, potassium, and selenium. Although they are mostly carb-free, you need to understand that the carbohydrate content varies for different kinds of seafood. For intermittent fasting, here is carb count for every 100-gram serving of specific shellfishes:

- **Clams:** 5 grams

- **Mussels:** 7 grams

- **Octopus:** 4 grams

- **Oysters:** 4 grams

- **Squid:** 3 grams

## *Smoothies*

A registered dietitian and natural foods chef based in New York named Miranda Hammer said that the key to making things healthy is striking the right balance of vegetables, fruits, protein, and fat. "The smoothie is a really great way to get all those foods in your body," she added. Creating homemade smoothies that are packed with fruits and vegetables, therefore, can be a great source of energy and give you different essential nutrients. Furthermore, smoothies have a lot of health benefits and seem trendy for people who are on a diet. They are also often given a vital part when it comes to cleansing and detoxifying. Thus, smoothies are essential when you are fasting.

## *Low-Carb Vegetables*

A nutritionist at Middleberg Nutrition in New York City whose name is Pegah Jalali once mentioned that low-carb vegetables are rich in fiber, vitamins, minerals, antioxidants, and many more. They also make a great vehicle for fats. The vegetables are considered a cornerstone of a low-carb diet, but one should take note of the correct varieties to consume. Overall, choose vegetables that are less sweet and starchy. The opposite of those are carrots, yams, beets, and turnips.

The foods and drinks mentioned above are probably the most recommended options if you need to top up your energy while fasting. Along with these are cheese, eggs, coconut oil, Greek yogurt, olive oil, berries, dark chocolate, and cocoa powder. It requires a strict amount of discipline and focus on your goal to realize why you are doing it. With moderation and self-discipline, you can enjoy these foods without suffering from the consequences that come with an ineffective weight-loss plan. Intermittent fasting comes with multi-health benefits, but eating something is needed to allow our body to function well throughout the fasting time. Furthermore, there are other recipes that you can prepare during your fast breaks to ensure the balance of nutrients in your body without compromising the essence of intermittent fasting.

William Cole, a Functional Medicine professor, recommends various recipes that you can try while fasting intermittently. In his segment, he has included simple meal preparations for your daily venture on intermittent fasting. For breakfast, for instance you can make a green smoothie. This can help to hype up your energy with a low-calorie drink rather than using a powdered fruit smoothie. You can use these following ingredients:

- 1 avocado

- 1 cup coconut milk

- 1 small handful of blueberries

- 1 cup spinach, kale, and orchard

If you plan to eat at lunch, you can prepare a healthy veggie burger to control your caloric intake and provide the energy that you need for the rest of the day. The recipe calls for:

- ½ pound ground grass-fed beef liver

- ½ pound ground grass-fed beef

- ½ teaspoon garlic powder

- ½ teaspoon cumin powder

- Sea salt and pepper to taste

- Cooking oil of your choice

Method:

1. Mix all ingredients together in a bowl and form the desired size of patties.

2. Heat cooking oil over skillet on medium-high heat.

3. Cook burgers in a skillet until desired doneness.

4. Store the burgers in a container in the fridge and use within 4 days.

If you are looking for a way to spice up your snacks, you can prepare cinnamon roll fat bombs. They are best eaten around 2:30 or 3 o'clock in the afternoon. The ingredients are:

- ½ cup coconut cream

- 1 teaspoon cinnamon

- 1 tablespoon coconut oil

- 2 tablespoons almond butter

Method:

1. Mix coconut cream and ½ teaspoon of cinnamon together.

2. Line an 8-by-8-inch square pan with parchment paper, and then spread the coconut cream and cinnamon mixture at the bottom.

3. Mix the remaining half a teaspoon of cinnamon with coconut oil and almond butter. Spread it over the

first layer in the pan.

4.  Freeze the snack for 10 minutes before cutting it into squares or bars.

There are also people who prefer to eat at dinner from 5:30 P.M. to 7:00 P.M. If you are one of them, you can prepare a salmon with veggies easily. Here are the ingredients that you need:

- 1-pound salmon or other fish of choice

- 2 tablespoons fresh lemon juice

- 2 tablespoons ghee

- 4 cloves garlic, finely diced

Method:

1.  Preheat the oven to 400°F, and then mix together lemon juice, ghee, and garlic.

2.  Place salmon in foil and pour the mixture over the top.

3.  Wrap the salmon with the foil and place it on a baking sheet.

4.  Bake for 15 minutes or until the salmon is cooked through.

5.  If your oven size allows it, you can also roast your vegetables at the same time.

# CHAPTER 8:

# EXERCISING AND
# INTERMITTENT FASTING

Exercise is a vital factor in your weight-loss journey. A regular workout routine matched with the power of intermittent fasting can help you maximize the benefits of both methods. When you stay physically active while fasting, after all, your body is forced to shed the fat that is detrimental to your health. It helps speed up the process of detoxification and autophagy as well, thus leaving your body rejuvenated, detoxified, and empowered. Despite that, too much exercise can affect you negatively. Like what we have discussed in the previous chapters, it is difficult to expend sugar and energy that your body does not have in the first place. According to researchers, when fasting and exercise are combined, it helps promote oxidative stress and prevent an increase of free radicals. According to Ori Hofmekler, a fitness expert, oxidative stress matters when it comes to maintaining your muscle mass. The condition not only makes you resilient to this acute kind of stress but also promotes the production of superoxide dismutase (SOD) and glutathione. Aside from that, it increase muscular capacity to utilize energy, generate force and resist fatigue. Thus, it is essential to schedule a daily workout routine to match your intermittent fasting plan.

When you exercise, though, you must eat food within 30 minutes after your workout. If you let the time go further than that, your body might break down and experience burnout, making you less inclined to finish your other activities.

Intermittent fasting is the process of limiting caloric intake through scheduling your meals at a certain timeframe. You can maximize the combined effects of fasting and exercise by scheduling your workout routine in the morning before you break your fast. This can help you increase your metabolism to a high degree. Not to mention, it is essential to kickstart your hormones and get you ready for a new day. Nonetheless, it feels equally important to listen to your instincts and be able to tell whether you need food before or after exercise.

In this chapter, I will be discussing the significance of maintaining a daily workout routine in lieu of fasting, as well as the types that you can employ as you move forward to a successful weight-loss journey. In the meantime, however, let me discuss the different forms of workout that you can use to complement intermittent fasting.

## TYPES OF EXERCISES

### Aerobics

Examples of this workout include swimming, dancing, and running, all of which are essential to strengthen your cardiovascular and respiratory systems. Apart from these, you can shed a tremendous amount of fat just by doing them from 15 to 30 minutes.

### Strength

This is one of the most common forms of exercise. However, it is more popular among men than women, considering the program consists of weightlifting, doing push-ups and crunches, and using bodyweight to build muscle mass. Too much strength exercise during fasting is not recommended for some people. Without enough energy reserve, after all, the workout may damage the body. As mentioned above, if you plan to do strength training during intermittent fasting, it is best to eat within 30 minutes after your routine. Listen to your body when it tells you to stop; never force yourself to continue when you are already weary or tired.

## *Balance*

This refers to the routines that help the body to acquire control and stability. A perfect example of it is yoga. This is the simplest, least extraneous, and most peaceful way to exercise and gain muscles. Even pregnant women are advised to practice it to increase their probability of having a normal birth. It allows for better relaxation and a stronger immune system. Imagine how much you can maximize its benefits when you combine this routine with intermittent fasting.

## *Flexibility*

This is the form of exercise that allows you to stretch your muscles to improve your range and joint motion. Examples of these exercises include tai chi, water dance, yoga, and many others.

## WHY SHOULD YOU EXERCISE?

Most people believe that when they are already fasting intermittently, they should no longer be required to exercise. Quite frankly, workout and fasting go hand in hand so that your well-being can improve. Remember that exercise is not merely about weight loss; it provides several advantages as well.

## 1. Strengthens Bones

Did you know that working out can increase your bone density and prevent osteoporosis? The latter is a condition in which the bones lose their density and are left to become weak and porous. It is most common among the elderly; that's why they are required to take a sufficient amount of calcium and maintain a regular exercise routine.

## 2. Prevents Cancer

Research has proven that exercise and fasting can reduce the onset of cancer among individuals.

## 3. Regulates Blood Pressure

As we have discussed earlier, fitness can promote the secretion of endorphins, which are essential when it comes to decreasing the level of cortisol in the body. If you have not noticed it yet, when people deal with an excessive amount of stress, they are more prone to having high blood pressure and hypertension, which can be dangerous for anyone.

## 4. Enhances Emotional Well-Being

Most people might not also be aware of it, but exercise can enhance your emotional health. Observe some individuals who are frustrated and depressed, for instance. They go to the gym instead of sulking in their houses and thinking about their day. A workout session can serve as a distraction to people who have a lot of thoughts that can cause distress. This process can help you obtain self-awareness and self-control. These are factors that are essential for maintaining a healthy psychological and emotional well-being.

5. Boosts Physical Health

Exercise, when combined with intermittent fasting, may allow you to maximize the benefits of holistic health. Together, they can strengthen the immune, cardiovascular, and respiratory systems. They can also inhibit the onset of stroke, atherosclerosis, apnea, and other diseases that you might acquire later in life.

## EXERCISING WHILE FASTING

After everything has been said and done, it is time to create your own workout routine to help you achieve your weight-loss goals. Remember that there is no specific time required for exercising as long as you have a regular way of doing it. If you feel like you are freer in the morning, you can workout for 15 to 30 minutes. However, if you are on a tight schedule during the day, you can do your routine before you go to sleep. Consider your daily activities while planning to avoid any time constraint that might stress you out more. Do not forget your situation and resources either. For instance, do you have a family to take care of? Are there possible distractions at home? Are you likely to exercise at the gym or home? If you're worried about the equipment needed for working out, you have nothing to fret about. There are exercises that do not require any tool except for your body weight. However, if you want to ante up your game, you might consider getting a gym membership and hiring a personal trainer. Be sure to inform whoever that individual may be that your fasting so that he or she knows what routines to suggest and ask you to avoid. If you choose to work out at home, you can utilize your gadgets to look for applications that can assist you digitally. You may also search for tutorial videos to watch; regardless if you are into Zumba or bodyweight training, you can always use the online experts' examples as a basis for exercising while fasting.

When you are a beginner when it comes to working out, you need to take things lightly during your first days of training, and then work your way up. Your body is very resilient. Even if you start at the low levels, it has the inclination to increase the intensity of the exercise as time passes by. Unknowingly, you will do more repetitions and sets than you have expected. From this, you will know that your exercise routine is totally worth it because it has significantly improved your stamina and agility in working out. Here are some tips to follow when exercising to lose weight.

1. Take note of routines that feel good to repeat.

I cannot tell you exactly what to add to your training program because we all have different preferences and body types. It is up to you to discover the forms of exercise that are fit for your body. In choosing these workouts, though, you need to make sure that you can execute the moves without causing injury on yourself. You must also consider the energy that you have left after fasting. Do not strain your muscles too much either. Let your body start from the easiest routines and adjust to it before moving on to the next level.

2. Remember to hydrate yourself every now and then.

If you want to break a sweat, you are going to need lots of water to facilitate the process of detoxification. This way, you can hasten your metabolic rate, as well as the burning of fats.

3. Learn to rest in between reps and sets.

Repetition is the number of times that you do a routine. For instance, 10 push-ups, 10 crunches or ten squats. A set, on the other hand, is the group of actions that you perform throughout the entire session. For example, one set may include 5 push-ups, 5 crunches, and five squats. You may say, "I did two sets of 15 repetitions of squats." That means that you have squatted 30 times. When you are in the middle of a workout routine, learn to rest your muscles every now and then or from 10 to 15 seconds after every action before moving forward to the next routine.

4. Do not exhaust the same muscles on the same day.

If you plan to start exercising now, you should decide on which muscle group to train first. Tomorrow, you need to choose a different muscle group, too. When you exhaust the same areas over and over, it may cause damage to the sheaths of muscles. Instead of having a lean muscle mass, its formation might become distorted and awkward to look at.

5. Perform warm-up exercises all the time.

This is one of the most important tips of working out: always learn to warm up for at least 5 minutes before an exercise to avoid any injury. This may include stretching, walking, or even cycling.

6. Utilize your distractions perfectly.

If you're so distracted with a television for the radio, for instance, you can use this to pump up your energy every time you are working out. It can also be a makeshift timer for your routines. If you get bored while doing so, you can turn on the TV and watch a show while performing the exercises. Meanwhile, when using the radio, you can use the songs or programs as cues for your routines. It may seem simple, but it is a very helpful tip to keep any distractions from getting in the way of your weight-loss goals.

# CHAPTER 9:

## EFFECTS OF HAVING MALNUTRITION

People who pride themselves in being too fat often say, "This is who I am. Why should I change it?" Others quip, "I am contented and proud no matter what the weighing scale says." Although there is nothing wrong with accepting who you are, there is a deeper reason why you need to lose weight, especially if you have gone beyond your normal body mass index (BMI).

BMI is the measure of your body fat. If the value is normal, it means that the ratio of your height and weight is ideal. This usually entails that you are a healthy person with a healthy lifestyle. However, if your BMI is outside the healthy weight-height ratio, you are either malnourished or overweight, which can both lead to various diseases. When you fast, therefore, remember to check your body mass index regularly to avoid going below or above the normal value.

Before we start talking about malnutrition, though, let me discuss the essential fats that we need to clear out to prevent confusion and misrepresentation in the future. The first and most important term to recognize is adipose tissue, a.k.a. fat. This is the anatomical term for the loose connective tissues in the body that consist of adipocytes. Its role is to store energy in the form of fats that cushion and insulate the body. It also has four types, namely visceral fat, subcutaneous fat, fibrous fat, and cellulite.

**Visceral fat** is the kind of adipose tissue that is stored tightly between the organs in the abdominal cavity, including the liver, pancreas, and intestines. Too much visceral fat inside the body is the cause of a hard stomach (or "beer belly" to alcoholics). The more it accumulates, the more it pushes the abdomen outwards, which gives someone a remarkable gut. Luckily, for women, they are not as prone to storing visceral fat as men.

However, for us ladies, we are more prone to having **soft fat**, a.k.a. **subcutaneous fat**, which can be found close to the skin's surface. This kind of adipose tissue is very soft and rounded. Hence, its other term is "fluffy fat." The female hormones signal the body to hold onto these fats to prepare for several significant events such as pregnancy, menstruation, and puberty. This is the reason why we experience bloating and weight gain before any of them take place.

We also have **fibrous fat**, which is tougher and more difficult to get rid of than subcutaneous fat. One example of fibrous fat is the excess fat that shows around your bra. Due to the pressure from clothes, and other garments, fluffy fat becomes fibrous fats, making it challenging to burn and expend as energy for various forms of physical activity.

**Cellulite** is a term that most of us might have heard of. Did you know that 80% to 90% of women have cellulite in their system? These chains of adipose tissue accumulate in the bottom layers of the skin, and it worsens as people age. Cellulite is also known as the "orange-peel skin" because of its observable texture. It is usually found in the buttocks and thighs, but it can also occur in other areas. There are many factors that contribute to cellulite in the body. E.g., smoking, alcohol, lack of physical activity, tight garments and underwear, hormonal imbalance and genetics. Nevertheless, it doesn't mean that it cannot be fixed or prevented. We will get to that later.

## MALNUTRITION AND OBESITY

Malnutrition can entail different things, although most people only refer to it as the lack of nutrients in the body. In truth, the term has two classifications, namely undernutrition and overnutrition. The former means that your body is not getting enough healthy foods; that's why it leads to serious illnesses like stunted growth, eye problems, diabetes, and heart disease. When a person is undernourished, he or she is likely to have a weak immune system that's supposed to ward off even the weakest bacteria or virus there is. Other symptoms of this kind of malnutrition are: hollow cheeks, sunken eyes, swollen stomach, dry hair and skin, delayed healing of wounds, and constant fatigue. In addition to that, did you know that undernutrition can cause depression and anxiety? When the body does not get enough nutrients that aid the production of serotonin, the individual tends to develop these psychological disorders. Serotonin, which is also known as the happy hormone, is one of the most important neurotransmitters out there, along with dopamine (the pleasure hormone) and endorphins (the feel-good hormone). Anorexia nervosa and schizophrenia are also linked to undernutrition because of loss of appetite, purging, and starvation.

Undernourished individuals lack common nutrients and minerals such as Vitamin A, which is essential in maintaining perfect eyesight. Undernourishment can also lead to enlarged thyroid glands and decreased the production of thyroid hormones due to the lack of iodine. They are deprived of zinc as well, a mineral that is responsible for appetite, growth, and healing. Iron is essential for brain functioning, regulating body temperature, and avoiding stomach problems such as the Kwashiorkor disease. This condition is characterized by a severe protein deficiency as well, causing fluid retention and a protruding abdomen. This is common among children in Africa.

The most common causes of undernutrition include food insecurity, digestive problems (e.g., Crohn's disease), bacterial overgrowth in the intestines, and celiac disease. Excessive alcohol consumption is another reason for undernutrition in adults because the content of alcoholic beverages inhibit the intake of protein, calories, and micronutrients needed in the body.

## EFFECTS OF MALNUTRITION

In every social media platform, we can see reports about undernourished people. Sometimes, when we go outside our homes, it is inevitable to see at least one homeless person looking for food. There are families who cannot eat within a day because they lack the resources to purchase what they need for their families. We see them and often ignore them. We do not even know what it really feels to have malnutrition. So, to further understand the importance of a healthy body, let us take a look at some of the effects of malnutrition in a person.

## 1. Reduced muscle mass and low stamina

Malnutrition causes a person to be weak and fragile. You may find it difficult to perform regular activities and exercises because of it. When dealing with undernourishment, you may not have the energy and strength either to climb stairs, carry objects, walk far, and even stay awake.

## 2. Wounds take longer to heal

Lack of protein, vitamin C, zinc, carbohydrates, collagen, vitamin A, and other nutrients are needed for wound recovery. If you are malnourished, an injury takes more time to heal for you than for most people and might be subject to inflammation and infection.

## 3. Low immune system

Malnourished people easily get colds, cough, flu, and other illnesses because they lack the nutrients that boost their self-esteem.

## 4. Poor sex drive and fertility problems

When women try to conceive, it is important to develop a healthy body and change your lifestyle for the better. Without proper vitamins and minerals, this dream may be almost impossible for you to achieve.

5. Difficulty in staying warm

This issue is due to lack of muscle tissues to ward off the cold. Fats keep us warm, especially during the cold weather. One of the reasons why many people die during winter is that they lack of supportive fats that envelop their bodies.

## FACTORS CONTRIBUTING TO WEIGHT GAIN

Overnutrition, on the other hand, leads to overweight and obesity. People who are experiencing this condition are more likely to have inadequate intake of vitamins and minerals. For example, in a study of 285 adolescents, researchers have found that obese people have lower vitamins A and E at an approximate level of 2% to 10% than those with normal BMI. This is most likely because being overweight or obese is caused by too much consumption of processed, junk, and fatty foods with high calories but lacks the essential vitamins and minerals needed by the body. Apart from these, there are other factors that contribute to weight gain.

### *Developmental Determinants*

From the term itself, the developmental determinants of weight gain refer to the "big moments" in a woman's life. One common example is the prenatal stage of a mother. Researchers have proven that mothers who have been declined of food and starved at the beginning of the first trimester are more prone to develop obesity, diabetes, and hypertension in their later years. Having a low birth weight is also associated with higher visceral adiposity in life, and it comes with a greater risk of cardiovascular and respiratory diseases.

The postnatal stage is also a factor in gaining weight. After recovery, there are some women let themselves go into binge-eating unhealthy foods, thus increasing the probability of being obese or overweight. You may have seen some mothers to significantly bloat after giving birth because they claim that they "have no reason" to maintain their sexy figure. To them, all that matters is they give what their child needs no matter what the cost is. They forget their daily exercise routine and the importance of having an inadequate amount of rest, which are both associated with increased weight.

Adiposity rebound is one of the most common causes of being overweight among children between the ages 5 to 7, too. This concept entails the significant increase of adipose tissues in children as they grow older. Researchers claim that this stage is the peak of growth in the youngsters. It is observed to be the years where they are most active, curious, innovative, and experimental in their surroundings. In turn, they will need a substantial source of energy; hence, they feel the need to eat more. Researchers have proven that kids who experience an adiposity rebound at earlier ages are more prone to developing obesity later. As we can observe in our own children, they are less active in their toddler years, and they have a little exercise to help burn the energy consumed for the day. Early adiposity rebound is attributed to advanced muscle and skeletal maturity of the kids, as well as the high protein intake of the parents during pregnancy.

Adolescence is another developmental stage that contributes to weight gain. This is the phase where adipose tissue deposition increases rapidly for some people. In which case, when a lady in her pre-adolescent period has too much body fat, chances are, it can increase remarkably during adolescence especially, with all the changes in her lifestyle and diet. Some even go through puberty and compensate its effects through eating and slacking off, thus causing more fats to stay within their system.

Adulthood is also a phase when you can gain extra pounds. As you perhaps know by experience, most of us have been physically active as teenagers. But as we grow up, we experience a sudden decline in physical activity. Plus, there is a gradual decrease of metabolism at this stage, slowing down absorption and breaking down of nutrients in the body. There are instances, on the other hand, when you may be too active in sports and other physical activities until early adulthood. When you stop doing all of that, there is a great probability for you to deal with bloating, especially when a high amount of food intake is not a complemented by physical exercise.

### Genetic and Environmental Determinants

There are two factors that define the structure and personality of a person. Some studies that prove that the human genome is a significant factor for being overweight or obese. Researchers have found out that energy balance, metabolism, dietary components, and activity levels can be inherited from the parents. So, when a child is born in an overweight family, there is a huge chance that he or she might become one as well. Nevertheless, this should not stop you from trying your best to lose weight. Obesity might be in your genes, but it will not develop if you will not allow it to happen.

The second one is environmental factors. If you put yourself in a habitat where you can live a healthy lifestyle and prevent yourself from having obesity, then you are in a safe place. There is a concept in psychology called "learned helplessness," coined by Martin Seligman, to define people who have given up on their situation because they either are used to it or feel like they can never get out. This is characterized by low self-esteem, passivity, poor motivation, procrastination, and failure to ask for help. If you let yourself sink in this black hole, then you will not be able to make positive changes for your body.

A person's energy usage, which is also known as the energy expenditure, is divided into three main components, namely the resting metabolic rate (RMR), thermic effect of feeding, and energy expended for physical activity.

The resting metabolic rate is defined as the energy used or expended when a person is at rest, e.g., sleeping, sitting down, or doing other neutral tasks. When your RMR is too low, then there is a higher probability for you to be overweight and obese. The thermic effect of feeding, on the other hand, refers to the increase of energy expenditure after a meal is consumed. Lastly, the energy expended for physical activity, including involuntary movements, such as shivering, fidgeting, and posture control, is a vital factor to determine the weight lost and gained by an individual. When all of these factors are very low in rate, you are more likely to be overweight than not. You will need a strenuous amount of physical exercise and to pay more attention to their diet to solve this issue.

Smoking and alcohol also play a role in weight gain. Cigarette smoking gradually decreases the metabolic rate and limits food intake of a person. When you quit smoking out of the blue, the consequences fall back to gaining extra pounds. Meanwhile, did you know that excess alcohol in the body, when unused, gets stored as fat? This is the reason why drunkards develop what is commonly known as "beer belly."

There are also drugs that contribute to bloating and weight gain. Glucocorticoids, such as prednisone, hypoglycemic agents like insulin, and anti-allergens can have an impact on the matter. Other drugs, namely hormone therapy and contraceptives, anti-seizure drugs, antidepressants, and heartburn medication, may cause you to gain weight as well. Because these chemicals may contain stimulants that can hype your diet, your metabolism rate can decrease, thus preventing your body from burning sugars and calories at a higher pace.

# CHAPTER 10:

# INTERMITTENT FASTING

# WHILE MENSTRUATING

As much as we hate to have our period sometimes, it is a natural and necessary process that women deal with every month. We all know that menstruation occurs when an egg cell is not fertilized by a sperm cell. Despite that, some of us still do not know the main effects of menstruation on the body. In truth, it is a cleansing mechanism that flushes out toxins and other substances in the body. As you may have observed after a menstruation cycle, your skin becomes clearer and more refined than before. The reason is that the foreign bodies that we constantly take in are eliminated through the blood that we expel by menstruating.

However, we cannot help to think about the effects of fasting while you are on your period. Is it even okay to fast while menstruating, or do you need to stop for a while? What are the effects of fasting before and during menstruation? We need to know these things for sure.

According to experts, fasting is like menstruation, in the sense that they are both natural processes. There are times when women do not have an appetite before, during or after menstruating, depending on your body's mechanism. Furthermore, the two methods can cleanse and regenerate the system to make new cells. However, there are instances when women experience pain and difficulty during menstruation. Some even deal with hemorrhagic anemia, a condition that takes place due to excessive menstruation. If this happens, the situation might worsen if you still decide to continue fasting.

Let us take a look at the few people who believe in fasting - the Muslims. It is no secret that during Ramadan, they mostly fast and pray. Nevertheless, what will occur if a woman is on her period? Will she be allowed to fast? According to Rose Khan, a 20-year-old Muslim, the menstruating women are excused from fasting during this time. Since menstruation is already a form of cleansing - and a way to lose nutrients, for that matter - fasting might overdo the process. The Muslim folks believes that although it is sacred to fast during the holy month for them, they must always consider the safety of their people first. Hence, allowing the females to skip fasting while on the period is reasonable. It shows that they understand that some women experience heavy and painful menstruations; that's why they cannot fast even if they want to.

There are several factors that govern a woman's menstrual cycle. It includes stress levels, energy levels, nutritional intake, and caloric intake, all of which are affected by intermittent fasting. We have discussed that one downside of intermittent fasting is the cessation of the normal functioning of some organs. Doctors have reported as well that the women who fast may experience irregularities in their periods. The truth is that this usually happens when a person fasts excessively without guidance. Thus, it matters to carry over the procedures effectively to avoid these shortcomings.

Nonetheless, if you are determined to fast on your period, there is a way for you to avoid burnout and fatigue during those days. To ease your worries, you should know that there are some people who benefit from fasting while menstruating. In a certain study, women with polycystic ovary syndrome (PCOS) have shown that fasting during a period gradually decreases stress levels and has limited effects on follicle-stimulating and luteinizing hormones. For overweight and obese females, fasting during menstruation has also been reported to cause a significant weight loss and decrease the onset of inflammation in the body. Before you fast on your period, though, have yourself checked up first. As long as your OB-GYN doctor says that you are fit to fast, I do not see why you cannot do it. However, to apply intermittent fasting while menstruating, you are going to need a less extreme way to fast and lessen your caloric intake. As much as possible, avoid the fasting schedules that can deprive your body of nutrients and minerals. Stay away from routines as well that allow you to acquire hypoglycemia or low blood sugar. Apart from these, here are some tips to remember when you decide to continue fasting during your menstruation.

## HOW TO FAST WHILE MENSTRUATING

### *Rehydrate Your Body*

We have previously discussed the different beverages that you can drink to break your fast. It includes water, tea, and coffee. These liquids can help you boost the level of antioxidants in the body and cleanse away the foreign, harmful, and unnecessary substances that may be lurking in there.

### *Take Multivitamins*

Taking iron-rich vitamins can help you foster a more efficient menstrual cycle. To avoid anemia and other conditions, you need to have sufficient levels of iron and vitamins C and B-complex. These minerals will help you ensure that your energy does not fall short while fasting on your period.

### Listen to Your Body's Needs

Whenever your body signals you something, you should never ignore it. If it tells you that it needs a bit more sugar, it means that it needs as much energy it can get from foods. Give your body some time to revitalize and recharge during your period. Having more amount of sugar and calories in your body will not hurt your fasting protocol since the cycle will take care of these extra fats for you.

### Avoid Strenuous and Stressful Activities

To avoid menstrual cramps and fatigue, it is best to lay off difficult activities for the week until your body is strong enough to carry over these activities. If you want to exercise, you may do so as long as you know your body can expend the energy that you need for your activities. If you cannot, you can compensate for the lack of exercise by walking short distances or meditating.

### Keep Your Fasting Periods Short

When you are menstruating, you should avoid fasting for more than 12 hours. For a more efficient plan, you can choose the 5:2, 6:1 or 16:8 pattern, provided that your body has enough energy for your other activities.

# CHAPTER 11:

## INTERMITTENT FASTING

## FOR WOMEN OVER 40

Who said that women cannot fast when they go beyond the age of 40? I mean, a lean and healthy body is not limited to the young ones. They can also be acquired by our mothers, aunts, and even grandmothers. There are many people over 40 years old who have gained the body that they deserve to have. As we have discussed previously, there are various advantages of fasting that the ladies can follow, so you can achieve your fitness goals regardless of your age.

Detoxification is one of the effects of intermittent fasting that is needed by people over 40 years old, especially the women. Over the course of your lifetime, after all, your body has been subject to various environmental changes. You may have also been taking in several harmful substances that can affect the immune system and cause several illnesses as you grow old.

When you fast, they can reduce the effects of these environmental factors and cleanse the body from the inside out.

Autophagy is also a process that works best for women about 40 years old. As mentioned in the past chapters, it involves the destruction of worn-out and dysfunctional cells. During intermittent fasting, you are more likely to experience a positive change in your skin and hair, making it more supple, radiant, and beautiful from deep within. The same is true with your internal organs. As we all know, they are composed of cells as well. Effective intermittent fasting will allow these organs to rejuvenate and become as good as new. This fosters a stronger cardiovascular system, respiratory system, reproductive system, and digestive system. Not to mention, intermittent fasting can help you avoid the stressful circumstances that you might encounter during the menopausal stage. This process is extremely vital, therefore, to help your body regenerate the integrity of its internal aspects and make you healthier than ever.

For example, for women who have acquired bad habits such as drinking alcohol and smoking cigarettes, intermittent fasting allows the cells in your kidneys, lungs, liver, and heart to get better, unless the substances have caused enough damage to the organs to the point of no return. How amazing is it to develop a perfect and healthy body even at 40 years old?

Nonetheless, there are fasting disadvantages that you should know about at this stage. You might already be aware that as you get older, your immune system becomes weaker as well. This makes the body prone to several diseases such as cardiovascular disease, diabetes, osteoporosis, and many more. If you cannot obtain a sufficient amount of nutrients to ward off these kinds of illnesses, then you will be putting your body in grave danger. Before you engage in intermittent fasting at 40 or above, therefore, you should consult your doctor about it first. And if you are very much determined to try intermittent fasting at this age, there are some tips to remember to maximize the effects of this process.

## FASTING TIPS FOR WOMEN OVER 40 YEARS OLD

### *Ask Yourself Why*

There are a lot of people who remain skeptic when they hear about the magic of intermittent fasting as it can help someone lose weight and obtain a healthy body. As a woman over 40, you need to rethink your priorities, as well as decisions to engage in intermittent fasting before you start. Are you really ready for this? Why do you need this? What can you gain from it? After answering these questions honestly, you can get motivated to develop a healthy lifestyle as the time passes by. It allows you to have self-control and be able to ward off any temptation to overeat and try harmful activities. Without that, you are bound to fail in your attempt to acquire a healthy body. So, stay true to yourself. If you start intermittent fasting without commitment, you will only be wasting your time.

### Apply the Golden Rules of Weight Loss

The golden rules of weight loss at the age of 40 require you to eat less by cutting back your meal portions, aim to lose 1 to 2 pounds per week, and remember that skipping meals will mess with your metabolism. Ironic, isn't it? For younger people, it is totally normal to forgo breakfast or any other meal of the day to follow an intermittent fasting schedule successfully. However, for women who are aged 40 years old and above, skipping meals can totally cause a decline in your metabolism; that's why you should merely consume fewer calories in a more frequent manner. We will discuss it later in this segment.

### Rethink Your Nutrient Intake

Another tip for fasting when you are 40 years old is to always keep your carbohydrate intake in check. It is advisable to add more protein to your diet to avoid muscle loss, as well as speed up your metabolism. In your diet, you must have fruits and vegetables, as well as lean protein from Greek yogurt, eggs, chicken, and fish. Also, when you do grocery shopping, make sure to include whole grains, beans, and other healthy foods on your list. Furthermore, did you know that fats are essential to improve muscle mass and bone density? To do this without stripping the essence of intermittent fasting, aim for 7 to 10 grams of fat every time that you have it on the table. That is approximately about 1 ½ teaspoons of olive oil, ¼ of avocado, and two tablespoons of nuts and seeds.

### *Do Not Forget to Stay Physically Active*

As we have discussed in the earlier chapter, exercise and fasting are not bad at all together. To maximize the benefits of these two methods, you need to observe a regular routine every day. It doesn't matter what kind of exercise you do as long as it fits your body and will not possibly injure you. It can pertain to 15 or 30 minutes of walking every day or stretching in the morning; what matters is that you are moving and your muscles are working.

### *Eat Fewer Calories More Frequently*

Researchers have found that as a person grows older, their metabolic rate declines along with it. To slow down this process, it is recommended to eat fewer calories in a more frequent manner rather than eating foods with a high number of calories less frequently. The latter process is a common mistake when it comes to fasting. If you aim to speed up your metabolism and the process of autophagy, you are going to need a few calories in frequent doses.

## *Mind What You Eat*

There is a famous saying that goes like, "You cannot teach old dogs new tricks." However, I beg to differ. The human mind is resilient no matter how old a person may become. I genuinely believe that the more you are, the more you are granted with self-control. To maximize the effects of intermittent fasting, you are going to need to learn to say no to certain foods even if you enjoy them so much. In case you want to lose weight or develop a healthy body, you need to be more careful of what you eat, as well as watch out for those choices that give you heart disease, diabetes, and other related conditions.

## *Avoid Alcohol and Cigarettes*

Drinking alcohol and smoking cigarettes will nullify the true effects of intermittent fasting if you keep on doing them. As much as you love these activities, you have no choice but to quite on both for the sake of being healthier than ever. If you have been an alcoholic your whole life, it may be extremely difficult for you to abstain from these substance. However, little by little, if you gain a bit of self-control every day, you can ward off the temptation of drinking alcohol or smoking cigarettes. Think about your health 10 or 20 years from now. How sure are you that you have not developed lung cancer, liver cirrhosis, or other illnesses due to these vices around that time? This might be a hard pill to swallow, but you're not getting any younger. If you want to live longer, you're going to need to change your lifestyle not for your family or friends but for yourself. There is so much to live for and see in life. You wouldn't want to miss those golden years of yours when you reach 60 or 70. Other people love to go for a reason. They believe that the remaining years of your life are when you truly see the wonders that it can provide. Why should you miss that opportunity when you have the chance to reach it?

Plus, if you have a family, wouldn't you want to see your grandchildren grow and become successful individuals in the future? Wouldn't you want to experience them pampering you, taking you to places you have never thought you can go to, and eating food that you have never tasted in your life? These little things matter as you grow older. Nevertheless, as you do, I hope you don't get a lot stronger and wiser.

# CHAPTER 12:

# COMMON MISTAKES WHEN DOING INTERMITTENT FASTING

You must have known by now that intermittent fasting is a tricky method for losing weight. You need to discover what your body really needs in order to experience and maximize the benefits of the process. What's risky about intermittent fasting is that there are several ways to do it and that there is no better way to find out which one suits you until you try them all. I am sure that you must have chosen a specific kind of fasting, and I totally hope it works for you. Now that you have established your goals towards successful intermittent fasting, you are now ready to start your journey and make your first step. But before you do that, you must furnish this information within your mind to avoid any setbacks or shortcomings during your fasting periods. In this chapter, I will be discussing the common mistakes that people do while intermittent fasting, as well as its effects on the body.

## *Being Too Hasty in Making Decisions*

During the process of intermittent fasting, it is inevitable for people to feel like giving up. At times, they can no longer help but eat. The question underlying this problem is, "Are you sure that you cannot go any longer or is your drive making you say and think of these words?" This is one of the main reasons why I am promoting self-mastery and self-discipline. In order to engage in intermittent fasting and experience its effects fully, you need to be more committed to your chosen line of weight-loss method. Yes, when you are fasting, you will feel irritable, angry, depressed, and frustrated about your actions. Sometimes, you will even feel stupid for trying because you know deep inside that you cannot do it. Your mind will be scouring for reasons to stop. However, it is up to you if you let it stop you from losing weight and experiencing its various health effects. I cannot prevent it if you want to give up already; you make your own decisions. And as they say, "You are the captain of your own ship." But before you throw in the towel too soon, I want you to rethink your choices and remember why you started intermittent fasting in the first place.

## *Not Eating Enough*

There are people who do intermittent fasting as a form of starvation. To them, they lose more weight without eating at all. They just don't know how much damage they cause to their bodies when they do not eat enough or at all. The reason why people drink during fasting is to avoid stomach, circulatory, kidney, and liver problems. When the body lacks the things it needs to function, it may cause detrimental effects to your overall death. This is what you need to watch out for. The people who fast for 36 hours experience more than what you do, and they have a way to distract themselves during fasting hours. So, do not try eating like a bird unless you want to get yourself in trouble.

### *Too much or Too Little Exercise*

There is a rule called the 80/20 rule, which states that 100% of your progress relies on 80% diet and 20% exercise or physical activity. The 20% is a significant amount to maximize the effects of intermittent fasting in the body. However, make sure that you do not overwork yourself, especially when you are not getting enough energy from your fasting periods.

### *Forgetting to Drink*

When your body is in a fasting state, it starts to break down and destroy dysfunctional and worn-out cells. In order to make the process effective, you're going to need to flush these toxins out by drinking water or tea or any healthy beverage of your choice. It is actually advised to drink about 4 to 5 liters per day, considering most of it gets consumed during fasting hours. Furthermore, drinking such fluids is the only way to compensate for the nutrients and energy that are needed by the body to perform several activities while fasting. Some people who engaged in intermittent fasting have been reported to sweat more during their fasting hours as well; that's why you cannot be dehydrated at all.

## Forcing the Body to Fast

We have discussed earlier that there are people who are not advised to fast. When you are one of them, kindly stop forcing yourself to lose weight through fasting. I am sure that there are other ways to fulfill your need to lose weight and obtain a healthy body other than this method. If you insist on fasting, you will only be putting yourself in danger.

## Making Excuses to Eat Junk

People with no self-control will always find a reason to eat what they want even if it is not a part of their fasting schedule. When I told you to listen to your body, I wanted you to be honest about the things that you feel and not make up a reason to break your fasting schedule. When you start doing the latter, your mind will be accustomed to the thought that it is okay and that no harm will come to you. The truth is, after everything that you have been through, it shocks me to find out that you are willing to sacrifice your efforts just because of a temporary enticement. Remember that the most permanent thing in this world is change. You will not be fasting forever. Why can't you wait for the right moment to eat and do whatever you want? I just hope that when you start fasting, you will be serious about it. Or else, this book will be all for nothing.

## Obsessing Over Intermittent Fasting

Finally, it is a mistake to let yourself get too obsessed with the process. When you allow yourself to be that way, you start to become dysfunctional in other activities. Your mind will revolve around the thought of intermittent fasting, which can be dangerous to your health. Being obsessed with the method tends to make you overfast, overcompensate, and overwork. This can cause burnout and extreme fatigue - two situations that can lead you to a hospital. Furthermore, when you get too obsessed with the process, there is a great tendency that you might experience depression every time that you fail to follow one of your schedules.

Let me clear up one thing. It is possible to develop a sense of self-mastery over your eating and fasting hours. However, it is okay to slip up from time to time. Committing mistakes and experiencing failures are normal parts of life. It makes us all human. So, live your life to the fullest while using intermittent fasting as a way to improve your lifestyle, live longer, and enjoy more of life's bounties.

# CHAPTER 13:

# THE POWER OF THE MIND MATTERS

We have mentioned at the beginning that mindset is an important factor for successful intermittent fasting. This chapter is one of the most vitals segments since it discusses various ways to control your mind whenever you contemplate between eating and not eating. So, I would gladly talk about how you can train your mind to say NO to every temptation that you encounter in your daily life. If you are used to eating more than three times a day, for instance, it will undeniably difficult for you to comply at first to the fasting protocols. However, as you push yourself harder towards success, there is no turning back. Your mind will be trained to withstand any temptation no matter how delicious or aromatic the food in your surrounding may be. In order to gain full control over your mind and emotions, you need to understand your possible urges and the reasons why you feel the need to comply.

## *Obsession*

Constantly thinking about foods that you should not have can reel you into giving in to temptations around you. It becomes unhealthy for the mind and the body to be obsessed with only one thing. Sooner or later, this will start to make you dysfunctional as a person. Rumination is the number one key to failure not only in intermittent fasting but in all aspects of life as well. When you find yourself thinking of eating over and over again, you ought to find a way to distract yourself through productive means.

## *Seeking Out the Action*

Your body starts to crave for eating or drinking too much because your brain is hardwired into such an activity. In other words, it has become a hard habit to break. In these cases, you can try to compensate on similar but more healthy behavior. For example, your body is looking for food at around 10 in the morning, but it is not time to eat yet. Instead of taking in loads of food varieties, settle for beverages and workout. That way, you can find another reason to fast until the eating window starts. It makes your vision about losing weight more clearly and more achievable when you motivate your body to stay away from foods a little longer.

## *Compulsively Engaging in an Activity*

The main problem with other people is their lack of self-control. When somebody asks them, they eventually agree and forget about their long-term goals. For this case, I want you to set your priorities straight. Think about the consequences that your actions are going to bring. What will you feel after you have eaten with your friends? Who have you fooled? It is not your friends whom you keep fooling but yourself. I do not mean to be blunt, but you will not finish anything successfully without the essence of self-discipline. So, before you say anything to anyone, give yourself time to think twice. These activities are just preliminary and temporary goals. They cannot help you in the long run. Focus on the length of your objectives and who you want to be in the future. I hope it helps you find the control you have buried within.

## *Withdrawal*

When a person suddenly stops a recurring action, such as smoking, drinking, or eating from fast foods, it brings on issues like irritability, restlessness, and depression. Because of these feelings, you may become more inclined to give in to temptation; that's why you tend to seek out the same actions and get obsessed with getting back in the game.

## Lack of Confidence

Self-confidence is one of the key factors to uphold in every goal, especially when you are fasting intermittently. Just by thinking "I cannot stop" or "I will not be able to accomplish it," you are already sentencing yourself to failure. So, before you engage in intermittent fasting or any other activity, make sure that you are emotionally prepared beforehand.

## HOW TO HAVE SELF-DISCIPLINE WHILE FASTING

Now, I will be teaching you how to have self-discipline in the midst of a difficult challenge. Imagine this: you are invited to a party, and you have no choice but to say yes. At the gathering, there are food and wine. It is impossible to restrain yourself from all the drooling over the varieties laid on the table. They have even managed to make all your favorite foods. Your mind and body are scouring for a way to convince your mind to go through with it. However, you know that you should never let your emotions guide your actions. So, what will you do then?

First, I want you to close your eyes and breathe. You can go to the comfort room for a moment if you want to. From there, you need to visualize your goals clearly. What do you want to do? Do you want to eat? Why do you want to eat? The common answers are, "I want to try the foods because they seem so delicious" and "Forget intermittent fasting; I will only live once, and today is my cheat day" (even when it is not). It can also be, "I cannot take it anymore. My friends are eating, and it will be rude to say no when somebody offers me food!"

In reality, these are just made-up reasons from your subconscious that tells you that you should eat. When you give in to the temptation, it means that your emotions have more control over your mind, which should never be the case. When you let your emotions take control of who you are, there are various repercussions that you are inclined to face, such as poor decision making, lack of problem-solving skills, and cowardice. You will not be able to live your life to the fullest by being emotionally driven. It is just a made-up reason because they no longer have control over the thoughts instilled by their pleasure principle. You need to learn how to separate your rational objectives from your basic drives. There are many ways to think rationally and bury these emotions.

While you are in a private spot, close your eyes and breathe deeply. Count from ten to one while thinking about other things, such as your breathing, what you are feeling, what you want to accomplish, and other stuff that may be standing in your way. Create a clear vision of your body and health goals as you breathe. Do not break your concentration. Just let the thought sink into your veins, giving you the power over your mind. Accept the emotions that you feel about not eating. Turn the frustrations into a ball in your mind and throw it away. Convince yourself that it is for the best. It is for your own good and benefit. Ask yourself, "Why should I waste a perfectly good streak right now?" Think about what you will feel if you eat. You will hate yourself for being too weak, too emotional. And you will regret having to binge-eat at the party.

Instead of looking inside yourself and searching for your emotions, ignore these drives and urges and turn it into control. Let your mind throw away the fear, pain, sorrow, and despair. Rather, see how much better you will be doing after you have finished your fasting routine. You want to wear your two-piece or one-piece bikini on the beach? Visualize that! Do you want to stop getting bullied because of your weight? Picture that out! Are you tired of all the names they have been calling you? Are you willing to accept that pain for the rest of your life? See, temporary pleasure does not account for a permanent and long-lasting change in your life. Do not be that person who lets herself commit a mistake and then wallows in regret after doing so. You know what they say: prevention is always better than cure. So, before you do something that you might regret, put yourself in a strong position where you can withstand the pressure of not eating.

## HOW TO SAY NO

The second issue is saying no to people who offer you food. The variety is already at your face, its aroma dancing around your nostrils like the devil in disguise. What do you do to say no so that no how much they offer to you, no matter how scrumptious they seem, you will not budge and give in? The main notion when you say no is the fear of offending the host and other guests for not eating. In truth, there is nothing to be afraid of or anxious about. After all, we are in the land of the free. As long as you pay your respect to everyone and converse with them graciously, you will not have a problem. They will not mind if you do not eat at all. If these people offer you food, they will not be offended when you say, "No, but thank you." If they ask you why, tell them that you are following a strict fasting schedule for health reasons. They will not demean you for that. In fact, they may even admire you for it. It takes courage to say no to a delicious meal. Just tell them you will only have tea or whatever drink they can offer. Granted, there will be individuals who will bash you for it, but who are they to think about? You are doing this for your own good, not theirs. When you are on the road to change, it is inevitable that some of your friends or family members will not be able to understand why you are doing this. Others might say that you have changed and that you have suddenly become a killjoy. But you need to make them realize that you are doing this to lose weight and improve yourself. You need to say no to the activities you have been excessively doing before, such as smoking, drinking alcohol, and even doing drugs. The hardest part is that intermittent fasting makes you say no to food. Do not expect everybody to understand what you need to change for yourself and why you want to change it. The people who are right for you will understand no matter what you decide to do. They will care about you and perhaps even help you in your weight-loss journey.

Furthermore, some individuals take it as a challenge to say no to other people because they are shy or nervous of getting rejected by the society. If they only knew the underlying reasons why you are fasting, then they will realize how important and difficult it is. Ignore the naysayers, as Arnold Schwarzenegger has said a million times. Focus on yourself and your health instead. Who cares about what they think? As long as your friends and family support and accept you for who you are, you do not need to get approval from anybody else. To say no to a person, you actually need to use the word and not beat around the bush. Avoid saying "I am not sure" or "I will think about it." When you really want to commit to decline, you have to say the magic word 'no.' So, here are some of the proven ways to say it without offending anyone.

The first one is to use firm but polite alternatives for the word. Use sentences such as "I appreciate it, but no, thank you" with a smile. You can also use the words, "Not today" or "I'm sorry, but I cannot. I'm not really into it. I think I will pass." When they ask you why, it is best to reply with a quick and subtle answer. If you go on and on about what you want to do, chances are, the asker will find a way to convince you and make you say yes. Make excuses such as, "I have a lot on my plate right now" or "I am too busy; I need to do a lot of things." Then, end your statement with another statement to change the topic or end your conversation by saying you have to go. You do not have to have an elaborate excuse for doing what you want. As long as you have made them understand that you want nothing to do with those activities, then you are good to go. When they ask you about it even more and try to reel you into agreeing, do not hesitate to say no as much as you can. Be as firm yet polite as you can be. No further reasons. However, there are instances when people can be very persuasive. So, before you get second thoughts into sticking with your intermittent fasting plan, think of the most rational explanation to tell them – something that they will believe and understand.

In other occasions, jokes work better than excuses. They won't even know that you are indeed joking. For example, when you are offered to eat at a party, you can just say, "No thanks, I am on a diet." Chances are, they will react in disbelief because of your statement. You already know what is in their minds. You can just manipulate them by saying,

"I'm already overweight, I need to trim down fats" confidently. Why? Because it is the most rational reason for saying no. They will even push you to do better. If they ask you about it, then you can tell them about your methods - no more, no less. Maybe by doing so, you will be helping other people in staying fit and healthy as well.

There is a phrase that defines most people nowadays that is known as "disease to please." This concept defines people who do their best just to belong in a group. If it means saying yes to everything and breaking your values and vows, they will take it, especially when it grants them fame. People in this generation believe that fame is a new source of power. Strangely enough, to win the hearts of people easily, you need to be famous. Even in politics, winning is not defined by your political platform but your popularity among the people. This is the concept that you should totally avoid not only for the sake of your health but also for the sake of your psychological well-being. You do not have to please everyone. You do not have to say yes to everything. You only need to be yourself, and you will get through life with flying colors. Think of it this way: when you have the disease to please, you might jump off the cliff the moment your friends decide to do it. You will ruin your life just to be "in." Is that the lifestyle you have always dreamed of as a child? When you are on the road to a successful intermittent fasting plan, you are not only training your mind to say no to food. You are training yourself to say no to every unhealthy activity there is in the world. And by committing to this venture and making it a habit, you can change not only your lifestyle but your way of thinking as well.

You know your friends so well, so you can tell which one of them is a serial asker and good persuader. It is always best to ignore them and avoid getting in contact with them, especially when you know there are significant events coming up. You can say no even when they have not asked you yet. This concept is known as crystal balling. If you ever get into the topic with something you want to decline to, you can call ahead of time and avoid any more persuasions by saying no. You can then say, "I'm sorry but I do not have enough money to go" or "My mom and I have plans for the weekend, so I cannot go." If you want to be softer in your approach, you can say, "I wish I could go, but I already made plans with some of my other friends this weekend" or "I wish I could go, but I already spent my cash on something else." "It is an honor. But..." could also be a phrase to start it off, especially when you are dealing with respected people in the society. White lies cannot hurt anyone, especially when it is for your own good.

If you are feeling uncomfortable and unconfident about yourself, you tend to be less assertive. But this should not be the case. Overweight or not, you have a reason to believe and stay confident about your talents and yourself. You need to be confident about the magnificent powers you are showing to the world by deciding to fast just so you can have the body you have always wanted. If that is not enough to boost your self-esteem, think of the successes you have had in your life. I am sure that those experiences can account for your unique abilities and personality as an aspiring human being. On the road to holistic change, you are going to need assertiveness. Do not let other people push you around like you are a child. You have your own decisions to make. You have your own battles to fight, including your goal to have a healthy body and a healthy lifestyle. So, when you talk to people, try to assert yourself more. What do you want? What don't you want? It is time to change the era of always being the second choice, the one who is pushed around. You are a beautiful and amazing person. Do you know that? It is time to learn how to become more mindful in the midst of peer pressure, anxiety, and belongingness in the community.

Now that you know the many ways to say no to many people around you, it is time to apply what you have learned. Practice makes perfect. The hardest part of declining to do your beloved activities is the feeling of being left out. Think of it this way: once you have regained your beautiful or healthy body, you can finally do whatever you want. Since we have discussed the various kinds of fasting, maybe you can employ some of the methods to give time for your activities and food. But for now, finish your 30-day challenge. Increase the time you need until you gain a healthy lifestyle you have always needed if possible. Think of those declines and missed opportunities as an inspiration to look forward. You just have to tell them, "Not now."

## HOW TO GAIN UNSTOPPABLE SELF-DISCIPLINE

Furthermore, it is important to employ the best methods to have self-discipline in everything you do. To maintain the right hours for eating, fasting, and exercising, you are going to need to train your brain as a ticking clock. It needs to be wired up in the sense that you are given an alarm clock from within. In this way, you will not miss your meals, eat while you fast, deprive yourself of sleep, and be unable to maintain a regular physical exercise. Without further ado, here are some techniques to acquire unstoppable self-control.

### *Create a Mantra*

Whenever you are unconfident about fasting, it is best to create an early morning mantra that starts with "I am." If you really aim to have a healthy and beautiful body, you can say, "I am strong enough to withstand any temptation today. In a few weeks, I will have the body I deserve to have." In cases where your self-discipline is challenged, you can close your eyes and say, "I am in control of my emotions and impulses. No person can command me of what I can do."

Repeat these mantras ten times or more, whatever you see fit. But you still need to claim it and believe that you can do what you are talking about. Otherwise, your mantra will be all for nothing. Let it sink into your mind and heart. As it does, you are left with a burning fervor to carry over your plan.

## *Write in a Journal*

A lot of people remain skeptic about writing all your thoughts and feelings in a journal. They say that it is a waste of time and energy because it does not do anything. On the contrary, journal writing is a very effective way to monitor your thoughts and feelings. It will be like giving yourself a pep talk whenever you feel like you are about to give up. Journal writing is a proven-and-tested method to pour down your feelings and feel good about yourself. Another fun fact is that this method actually helps in disciplining the mind. How do you ask? Writing entails focus and concentration. When you write in a journal, you are forcing your mind to dig deep within your level of subconscious and write everything you can think about in an orderly fashion. If you try this method, you can see a dramatic change in the way you organize your thoughts and control your emotions. Focus is the key, and this is one way you can train yourself to acquire it.

## *Practice Mindfulness in Everything*

Mindfulness is defined as putting yourself in the moment and being aware of your environment. For instance, when you are aware of how, what, and why you eat, not only will you be able to enjoy a perfectly good meal but you will also practice control over your eating habits and methods. Think of it this way, when a person does not emancipate mindfulness during mealtime, you tend to stuff any food on the table in your mouth. You cannot pay attention to the leptin hormone signaling your body that it is already time to stop eating. You can observe that in people who watch the television while having a meal as they tend to be more obese than others who stay away from such distractions. That is because they merely focus on what they watch and not on their food intake.

## *Learn to Rest*

People tend to be more emotional when they are restless. Imagine working graveyard shifts. Or, if you know someone who is totally restless, you know that they can be very irritable, angry, and dreadful. This is the reason why people easily give up. They feel tired in dealing with countless problems. When you are starting to feel this way, you should find a way to relax. When it is time for a break, get up from your chair and stretch or talk to your colleagues. Do not bring your work home if possible as well. Likewise, do not bring your family problems in the office. Learn to deal with things one at a time and try not to pressure yourself with everything else. When it is time to sleep at night, it is best to doze off for 7 to 8 hours to prepare yourself for a new day. Sleep and rest are known to rejuvenate the brain and body. They can put everything back in a state of balance along with all the chemicals and hormones. Finally, you are less stressed and less agitated when you wake up.

### *Share with Your Friends and Family*

This is a very important method to increase your social support. When you have enough people to keep you motivated towards your growth and improvement, they will be more than happy to get you through your ordeals and trials. Ask them to help you deal with any temptation and not to mock you while you are trying to stick to a diet. Get their assistance to stay on the right track as well by lifting up your spirits when you feel down and encouraging you to become stronger. You will find yourself more motivated to continue on your venture and be more successful in reaching your goals.

### *Find New Hobbies*

Hobbies are nice ways to get you distracted from food urges and frustrations. Boredom is one of your worst enemies when you are trying to fast. There are instances when people get too preoccupied on their thoughts and negative feelings when they feel bored. It's not that they are want to break their fasting, but they have nothing else to do. Thus, they are tempted to eat. We can observe several people who are inclined to eat whenever they get bored, so it is important to look for various things to get your mind off of the urge to eat, especially when you are with your friends and family.

## Be Socially Involved

It is possible to look for organizations that support the cause of fasting in society. For this matter, you can learn a variety of methods on how you can venture into intermittent fasting more successfully. Plus, if you find people who will push you and motivate you towards fasting, you will be more inclined to eat only as scheduled. When you stay active in this group, you will realize that there are people with more problems than you. By talking to them, you can learn from their experiences and gather a hack or two from their wisdom.

## Remove All Temptations

If you want to successfully accomplish your goal towards weight loss, get rid of anything that can tempt you into binge-eating. This includes emptying your refrigerator and cabinets of junk food and other unhealthy foods. Instead, fill it with tea, coffee, healthy beverages, and other liquids for rehydration. Whenever it is time to eat, avoid oily foods as much as you can and settle for vegetables and fruits for better effects.

## Don't Wait for It to Feel Good

One of the many reasons why people give up on intermittent fasting is that they do not feel good about the method. Well, nothing really feels good in the beginning, especially when you are trying to change your former habits. After all, when people start to quit alcoholism and smoking, the start is always rocky. There will be withdrawal and perhaps even depression to deal with at times However, if you are committed to doing something positive for yourself, do not wait for it to feel good. It only gets better after a few days, weeks, or months. As we have been reiterating, do not let your emotions take control over your mind.

## Learn to Schedule

When you have a poor sense of time, you better use an alarm to signal whether it is time to eat or not. Make a time frame for your workout routine as well. These things are important in slowly building a good habit that you can use in a lifetime.

## Don't Be Too Hard on Yourself

At the beginning, it is inevitable to deal with failures and mistakes. But the mindset to successful fasting is not built overnight. You need to learn to forgive yourself and move forward. Otherwise, you will be stuck and feel depressed and anxious every bit of the way. You have all the time in the world to restart and retrace your steps. You should not feel too guilty when you fail on the first days of your intermittent-fasting sessions. Just promise yourself that whenever you slip up, you will never cease to get back up and keep trying.

## *Learn to Give Rewards*

There is a concept in psychology called operant conditioning. Much like intermittent fasting, it is a method that has been around for centuries. Coined by B.F. Skinner in his early work between 1890 to 1930, operating conditioning ran supreme among many methods for behavior modification. It was based on Thorndike's Law of Effect, but with a little reinforcement. Skinner discovered this idea when he conducted an experiment on rats. He placed two levers in a box; when pulled, one would cause an electric shock, while the other would dispense pellets for the rats to eat. He found that the rodent avoided the electrocution lever and focused on pulling the one that would give them food. This concept can be applied to us humans in an effective fashion as well. When a person's mind is hardwired to think that a successful and good action constitutes a reward, you are likely to repeat the action again.

You can employ this method to train your mind and gain self-control while fasting intermittently, of course. You can reward yourself after a day of fasting efficiently by eating something that you love once it's time to break your fast. Better yet, you can give yourself something that you have always want to have after completing a whole week of successful fasting. When your brain starts to associate a positive thing with the practice, you are more likely to accomplish this goal one way or another despite the challenges it comes with.

# CONCLUSION

Intermittent fasting is not just a hobby that people try for fun. This is a proven method that will allow you to start living healthier. Intermittent fasting was first introduced by the father of medicine, Hippocrates, and had been in the minds of people for generations. Many other proponents of science have also become advocates of this practice. From their studies, they have found that intermittent fasting is not only used for weight-loss purposes. The truth is, weight loss is only a bonus. Intermittent fasting was initially known to prevent cardiovascular disease, respiratory issues, diabetes, promotion of growth, and longevity. Imagine how healthy your body is going to be after finishing the 30-day intermittent fasting challenge.

Sadly, there are people who are not recommended to try fasting. They are the ones with depression, anorexia, and even a baby on the way. However, if you have the opportunity to grab this method and commit to it, you will not regret engaging every moment towards intermittent fasting. Sooner than later, you will find yourself in the brink of a healthy lifestyle, equipped with an alert mind and a strong body. Who said you cannot regain a sexy body after bearing three children? Who said you cannot have a healthy lifestyle when you reach 40 or 60 years old?

All it takes is a whole lot of commitment, confidence, and self-discipline. These three are the main components of a successful intermittent fasting routine. Without any of them, your journey is bound to cease and fail. It is not easy to lose weight - that is a fact. There will be people who might demean you, bully you even more, and doubt every bit of your spirit. So, you need to be ready to deal with them. Never listen to naysayers and negative thinkers; instead, surround yourself with individuals who will love, accept, and support you in every venture that you choose. Your real friends and family will be happy to hear that you are doing something to improve yourself. The rest might undermine you because of it, but they should not matter anyway. As we have said earlier, you are not doing this for them. In fact, you are doing it for yourself. Think of the long-term effects of your intermittent fasting. Soon, you will be able to wear that sexy dress in the store and flaunt your body that has become healthy both inside and out.

I admire people with such grit and to change their bad habits wholeheartedly. They are willing to sacrifice their old hobbies for the betterment of their heart, mind, and soul. If you have read this book from cover to cover, it means that you have taken the first step towards having a successful life, and I want to congratulate you for it. It is not easy to put in so much effort in a book when you can just do other things. I hope that I have motivated you to become a stronger, fuller, and healthier woman. Always remember that you are beautiful. You are unique. You have spectacular talents. Let this book be a beacon towards a healthy mind and body. This way, you can imagine being on the front porch of your home, getting ready for work or school, and feeling confident as ever. You are now looking forward to meeting other people because you know all the positive changes that you have undergone internally are now visible externally. You no longer have to suffer the endless name-calling from ill-meaning people. You no longer have to endure the stares at restaurants, buses, and trains. You are now a changed woman, holistically speaking. Not only have you developed a healthy lifestyle but an amazing mindset as well. That is what intermittent fasting can do to you.

# BIBLIOGRAPHY

Australian Professional Skills Institute (2016). 7 time management tips for students. Retrieved from https://www.apsi.edu.au/7-time-management-tips-students/

Barnosky, A., Hoddy, K., Unterman, T., & Varady, K. (2014). Intermittent fasting vs daily calorie restriction for type 2 diabetes prevention: a review of human findings. Retrieved from https://www.translationalres.com/article/S1931-5244(14)00200-X/abstract

Bilich, K. (n.d.). 10 benefits of physical activity. Retrieved from https://www.parents.com/fun/sports/exercise/10-benefits-of-physical-activity/

Brazier, Y. (2018). Measuring BMI for adults, children, and teens. Retrieved from https://www.medicalnewstoday.com/articles/323622.php

Campbell-Avenell, Z. (2016). 49 ways to say no to anyone (when you don't want to be a jerk). Retrieved from https://www.careerfaqs.com.au/news/news-and-views/how-to-say-no-to-anyone

Charkalis, D. (2018). 13 dos and don'ts of intermittent fasting. Retrieved from https://www.livestrong.com/slideshow/1008373-master-fast-dos-donts/?slide=1

Cole, W. (n.d.). Intermittent fasting: A complete guide to benefits, diet plans & meals. Retrieved from https://www.mindbodygreen.com/articles/intermittent-fasting-diet-plan-how-to-schedule-meals

Crosta, P. (2017). Everything you need to know about cellulite. Retrieved from https://www.medicalnewstoday.com/articles/149465.php

Donelly, C. (n.d.). The do's and don'ts of intermittent fasting [Slideshow]. Retrieved from https://www.sharecare.com/health/diet-nutrition/slideshow/the-dos-and-donts-intermittent-fasting#slide-1

Fielding, S. (2019). Wondering why your beer belly is hard? Here are 5 possible causes. A rock-hard stomach isn't always a good thing. Retrieved from https://www.menshealth.com/weight-loss/a19543924/abs-diet-hard-belly-fat/

Foundation Education (2016). 5 essential self-management skills. Retrieved from https://www.foundationeducation.edu.au/articles/2016/10/5-self-management-skills-you-need-to-win-at-life

Fung, J. (n.d.). Fasting – A History Part I. Retrieved from https://idmprogram.com/fasting-a-history-part-i/

Gould, H. (2019). This explains so much: Turns Out we all have 4 different types of fat. Retrieved from https://www.byrdie.com/how-to-lose-fat

Gunnars, K. (2017). What is intermittent fasting? Explained in human terms. Retrieved from https://www.healthline.com/nutrition/what-is-intermittent-fasting

Greenlaw, P. & Greenlaw D. (2016). The history of dieting and weight loss: It started 2,300 years ago with the Greeks. Retrieved from https://www.christianpost.com/news/the-history-of-dieting-and-weight-loss-it-started-2300-years-ago-with-the-greeks.html

Harris, S. (2018). What happens if you fast for a day? Retrieved from https://www.medicalnewstoday.com/articles/322065.php

Harvard Health Publishing. (2017). Not so fast: Pros and cons of the newest diet trend. Retrieved from https://www.health.harvard.edu/heart-health/not-so-fast-pros-and-cons-of-the-newest-diet-trend

Holmes, P. (2010). The different types of fast. Retrieved from https://www.crosswalk.com/faith/women/the-different-types-of-fasts-11626299.html

Institute of Medicine (US) Subcommittee on Military Weight Management. (2004). Weight management: State of the science and opportunities for military programs. Washington D.C: National Academies Press. Retrieved from https://www.ncbi.nlm.nih.gov/books/NBK221834/

Jarreau, P. (2018). Your menstrual cycle on intermittent fasting. Retrieved from https://lifeapps.io/fasting/your-menstrual-cycle-on-intermittent-fasting/

Koman, T. (2018). 10 celebrities who swear by intermittent fasting. Retrieved from https://www.delish.com/food/g22617665/celebrities-intermittent-fasting/

Land, S. (2018). 15 different types of intermittent fasting and their benefits. Retrieved from https://siimland.com/15-different-types-of-intermittent-fasting-and-their-benefits/

Lefave, S. (2018). 8 major mistakes people make when intermittent fasting. Retrieved from https://whatsgood.vitaminshoppe.com/intermittent-fasting-mistakes/

Lewis, D. (2013). Explainer: Why do women menstruate? Retrieved from http://theconversation.com/explainer-why-do-women-menstruate-13744

Link, R. (2018). 8 health benefits of fasting, backed by science. Retrieved from https://www.healthline.com/nutrition/fasting-benefits

Lizzy Loves Food. (2019). My 30 days on intermittent fasting results. Retrieved from https://lizzylovesfood.com/30-day-intermittent-fasting-results/

Lowery, M. (2017). Top 5 intermittent fasting mistakes. Retrieved from https://2mealday.com/article/top-5-intermittent-fasting-mistakes/

Maternity Comfort Solutions. (2018). 7 intermittent fasting hacks to lose the baby weight. Retrieved from https://maternitycomfortsolutions.com/7-intermittent-fasting-hacks-for-losing-the-baby-weight/

McLeod, S. (2018). Skinner – Operant conditioning. Retrieved from https://www.simplypsychology.org/operant-conditioning.html

Mercola. J. (2013). Should you eat before exercise? Retrieved from https://fitness.mercola.com/sites/fitness/archive/2013/09/13/eating-before-exercise.aspx

National Eating Disorders Association. (n.d.). Anorexia nervosa. Retrieved from https://www.nationaleatingdisorders.org/learn/by-eating-disorder/anorexia

Nursing Times. (2009). Malnutrition. Retrieved from https://www.nursingtimes.net/malnutrition/5001811.article

Pedre, V. (n.d.). Intermittent fasting can be dangerous for some people. Here's exactly what you need to know. Retrieved from https://www.mindbodygreen.com/0-29932/intermittent-fasting-can-be-dangerous-for-some-people-heres-exactly-what-you-need-to-know.html

Pique. (n.d.). What to drink while intermittent fasting. Retrieved from https://blog.piquetea.com/what-to-drink-while-intermittent-fasting/

Polevoi, L. (n.d.). 8 tips for effective time management. Retrieved from https://quickbooks.intuit.com/r/employees/8-tips-for-effective-time-management/

PTI. (2018). Here's why women gain weight after pregnancy. Retrieved from https://www.deccanchronicle.com/lifestyle/health-and-wellbeing/100718/heres-why-women-gain-weight-after-pregnancy.html

Rampton, J. (2018). Manipulate time with these powerful 20 time management tips. Retrieved on https://www.forbes.com/sites/johnrampton/2018/05/01/manipulate-time-with-these-powerful-20-time-management-tips/#733967a857ab

Randone, A. (2018). What happens when you get your period during Ramadan. Retrieved from https://www.teenvogue.com/story/what-happens-when-you-get-your-period-during-ramadan

Rettner, R. (2016). The 4 types of exercise you need to be healthy. Retrieved from https://www.livescience.com/55317-exercise-types.html

Romm, A. (n.d.). 7 steps to get over food cravings & gain control of your life. Retrieved from https://www.mindbodygreen.com/0-13876/7-steps-to-get-over-food-cravings-gain-control-of-your-life.html

Science Daily. (n.d.). Adipose tissue. Retrieved from https://www.sciencedaily.com/terms/adipose_tissue.htm

Skills You Need. (n.d.). Dealing with stress - Ten tips. Retrieved from https://www.skillsyouneed.com/ps/stress-tips.html

Smith, L. & Lunders, K. (n.d.). 20 weight loss motivation quotes that will empower you to keep going. Retrieved from https://www.womansday.com/health-fitness/womens-health/g3209/best-weight-loss-motivation/

Spritzler, F. (2017). 16 foods to eat on a ketogenic diet. Retrieved from https://www.healthline.com/nutrition/ketogenic-diet-foods

Steve. (n.d.). How to build your own workout routine. Retrieved from https://www.nerdfitness.com/blog/how-to-build-your-own-workout-routine/

Streit, L. (2018). Malnutrition: Definition, symptoms, and treatment. Retrieved from https://www.healthline.com/nutrition/malnutrition

Taylor, M. (2018). 9 things you must do to lose weight over 40, according to experts. Retrieved from https://www.prevention.com/weight-loss/a20465042/lose-weight-over-40/

Thompson, C. (n.d.). 7 types of fast. Retrieved from https://www.livestrong.com/article/520268-7-types-of-fasts/

West, H. (2019). How to fast safely: 10 helpful tips. Retrieved from https://www.healthline.com/nutrition/how-to-fast

Whiteman, H. (2015). Fasting: health benefits and risks. Retrieved from https://www.medicalnewstoday.com/articles/295914.php

World Health Organization. (2018). Obesity and overweight. Retrieved from https://www.who.int/news-room/fact-sheets/detail/obesity-and-overweight

# SUSAN KATZ

# Easy as Pie
# Keto Fasting Guide

Fast and Effective Weight Loss with Intermittent
Fasting + Keto Diet (A Beginner Friendly Guide
for Women)

SUSAN KATZ

# INTRODUCTION

So here we are then. You've probably picked up this book after your latest diet has failed. Or perhaps you're simply tired of what you see in the mirror every time you look. You feel sluggish, overweight, and a climb up the stairs gets you huffing and puffing like you're trying to blow someone's house down.

By this time, you've probably tried a few diets and perhaps even saw some fleeting success with some of them. However, you must have then run into what every dieter out there experiences: the plateau. After that initial burst of weight loss, nothing happens, and you remain the same, except you're now working twice as hard, counting your calories the whole way.

Oh yeah, there's the counting calories bit. All of a sudden, food isn't food to you; it's some combination of calories which causes you to think about all the time. Does this put me over my caloric requirement? Can I afford, calorically speaking, to eat this now? Will, I put on more fat if I eat this?

It's safe to say that no matter what your intentions were when you started, they've been completely subverted thanks to the demands your previous diets have placed on you. You started out wanting to look and feel good. Instead, all those diets have now made you feel like you're attempting rocket science while juggling two plates at the same time while riding a bicycle.

I'm here to tell you; all this is coming to a stop right now! That's right! This book has the solution you need, and while it will take some work on your part, I promise you that the results you will see will only spur you on to greater heights. Instead of pouring over all those before/after pictures you see on Instagram, you can now take your own!

Here's my pledge: within four weeks, you will see a leaner, fitter version of yourself in the mirror by following everything laid out in this book.

## SO HOW DO I ACHIEVE THIS?

Losing fat and getting healthy is a simple process that relies on two essential principles: Intermittent fasting (IF) and the Ketogenic diet. You've probably heard of these concepts before but even if you haven't, don't worry. This book is a thirty-day guide to fat loss, and along the way, you will learn all about these concepts and more importantly, how to integrate them into your life successfully.

You see, a lot of diets prescribe something without taking your lifestyle into account. Then, there's the problem of a lot of diets not suiting women. Women face particular challenges that men do not when it comes to fat loss. For one, it is tougher for women to lose fat as compared to men and secondly, we girls tend to second guess ourselves more than the guys out there.

In this book, I've put together both the concepts, with the science behind them, as well as actionable plans for you to get started immediately. None of what I've written in this book is pie-in-the-sky type thinking - it's real and practical. IF and Keto are the most powerful ways to lose fat and get healthy.

By combining them, you get to access the best of both worlds!

## WAIT, WHY SHOULD I LISTEN TO YOU ANYWAY?

That's a good question! After all, who am I to lecture you on how to do things? I don't have a string of letters after my name, and neither am I a sexy Instagram babe. No. What I am is a regular gal who went through what you're going through right now and struggled with the same issues that plague you at this moment.

I've never had a model like physique, despite craving one and trying my damnedest to eat as healthy as possible. It seemed like everything I did had just one effect, and that was to increase the size of my waist and put on fat in areas where people would immediately notice. I struggled with body image issues, and these ran so deep that even today, I occasionally struggle with insecurity as well.

Once I gave birth to my child, this problem only became worse. What with my already low self-esteem and the pregnancy weight gain, I felt a growing sense of dread during what should have been one of the happiest moments of my life. Once my baby was born, though, I had a choice to make. I could either set a bad example and resign myself to something I hated, or be active in showing my child how you're supposed to deal with problems.

I discovered the Keto diet, and initially, it didn't make much sense to me. After all, how does eating fat help you lose fat? I decided to try it anyway since I didn't have much to lose. I saw results immediately and began shedding weight. However, I was still struggling to nail my calorie counts, and it was becoming unsustainable. I could tell the progress I had made would soon vanish, and I would regress because the method I was using was unsustainable.

Then I stumbled upon intermittent fasting. On the surface of it, this seemed like another form of food torture, to be honest. Go hungry for sixteen hours a day? Only eat for eight hours? Then again, what did I have to lose? I plunged heart and soul into it. Well, IF turned out to be the easiest thing I had ever done.

I found that my natural eating pattern, indeed the pattern for most of us, follows what IF prescribes. With a few barely noticeable adjustments, I was able to not only follow my plans but even ditch counting calories! That alone made me jump for joy.

Along the way, I also discovered the additional benefits of becoming healthier, and to this day, I continue to follow what's written in this book. There is no further information you need or something special you have to do to achieve the same results. It's all in here!

## SO, YOU'RE SAYING IT WORKS?

Absolutely! Once you follow this diet plan, you will see the fat melt right off your body. That's not an empty promise; it's merely the result of you reconnecting with the way human beings are supposed to eat! IF has several proven health benefits and has been practiced since ancient times (Gunnars, 2017).

IF increases your cellular level inflammation, possibly reverses Type 2 diabetes, lowers your blood sugar and insulin levels, and stimulates autophagy (Gunnars, 2017). Meanwhile, the keto diet is no slouch either. Along with the usual effects such as fat loss and increased energy, the keto diet also helps reverse Type 2 diabetes and is prescribed for many Type 1 diabetes patients as well (Gunnars, 2017).

In addition to this, it helps increase the good cholesterol within you and reduces the bad cholesterol, along with lowering your blood pressure (Gunnars, 2017).

If none of this convinces you, well your body's improved and sexy appearance will. I mean, it works for Beyonce, Nicole Kidman, Hugh Jackman, and Jennifer Lopez, so why wouldn't it work for you?

You will also experience the side effects of becoming healthier as I did. Your skin will look better, your overall appearance will be more pleasing, and your mood will be a lot better, thanks to having energy more often. No more huffing and puffing up the stairs!

## A COMMITMENT

Let me repeat this: By following the steps outlined in this book, you will not only become and feel healthier, but you will also have your friends come up to you and ask "What the f*ck have you been doing?!"

You will love the new you that appears in the mirror and will have both mental and physical energy as you go about your day. At first, it will seem counterintuitive, but I will show you proof of this working, in addition to what I've already shown you.

Best of all, I've given you a simple and easy to follow plan born out of my own experiences and the mistakes I made. This book is a practical, step by step plan which you will have no problems implementing in your life, and in a month's time, you will notice visible results!

So stop hating yourself and take action! There's no time like the present - indeed, it is the only time available to us. The steps outlined in this book require discipline, but this isn't some Navy Seal-like determination that's being asked of you. No, everything within this book is easily achievable by you, and you already have everything you need to succeed.

Best off all, it doesn't matter whether you're looking to lose five pounds or a hundred and five pounds, the solution is the same! In fact, the more weight you have to lose, the better this method works! You will be combining two of the most potent fat burning tools out there, and you will inevitably become healthy and achieve what you want.

So let's start then, shall we? Are you ready to change your life? Let's get into it!

# CHAPTER 1:
# WHY INTERMITTENT FASTING+KETO
# WORKS BETTER...MUCH BETTER

Some of you will be familiar with intermittent fasting and keto as separate concepts, while some of you won't. This chapter is for the latter group, and I'll talk about how IF as well as the ketogenic diet, impact fat loss and overall health. If you're already familiar with this topic and want to get into the nitty-gritty, please feel free to skip ahead to the chapter you wish to learn about, if not, let's get into it.

Fasting, in some form or another, has existed since ancient times as a method to treat disease as well as manage overall health. While a majority of the ancient techniques prescribed fasting periods of a day or sometimes more, intermittent fasting is a scientifically backed approach that removes the guesswork from the process of fasting.

To understand how the ketogenic diet can incorporate within its framework, we need first to understand what intermittent fasting is all about.

## INTERMITTENT FASTING

IF has been a fitness trend for a while now, but unlike most trends, this actually works. When your goal is to burn fat, it is your diet that plays the lion's share of the role in the process. With dieting, restrictions comes a variety of permutations and combinations that you need to take into account, and this often complicates things.

You've probably experienced this already with your last diet. The question of what to eat suddenly became a valid and, in some cases, terrifying experience. As you progressed along with your previous diet, the fear of eating the wrong thing would have intensified. A lot of dieters report such feelings when it comes to any diet regimen.

The easiest way to control what you eat is to do what is easily repeatable. In other words, the less you need to think about something, the easier it is to turn it into a habit. Think about it: Do you have to think about tying your shoelaces? No. It's deeply ingrained in your mind.

Similarly, your aim with dieting should be to simplify it as much as possible so that it is easier to adopt into your lifestyle. That's where IF can help.

## *Benefits*

While fat loss is a natural side effect of intermittent fasting, its health benefits go well beyond just that. Here is a small sample of benefits that IF provides.

Autophagy: Autophagy is the process by which cells clean themselves of harmful protein buildup. Thanks to the fasting portion of IF, cells initiate this process. A study conducted in 2010, which aimed to measure the rate at which Autophagy begins, concluded that the number of vesicles per cell (which is a measure of the autophagous response) increased within twenty-four hours of food restriction (Antunes et al., 2018).

Furthermore, autophagosome characteristics are also detected with an increase in the cell area, perimeter, and other physical changes. After forty-eight hours, these characteristics only increased. The results were validated against standard characteristics observed through electron microscopy methods, and thus, the results were deemed valid.

In other words, the biological markers of Autophagy increased significantly.

Metabolic Rate: Fasting intermittently increases our body's metabolic rate, which in turn causes us to burn more food more efficiently and aids in fat loss, depending on the composition of our diet. A study in 2000, aimed at observing the effect of short-term starvation in lean, healthy men and women, found that energy burned while resting increased significantly from the first to the third day (Zauner et al., 2000).

Also, the concentration of norepinephrine increased as well accompanied by a decrease in serum glucose. Insulin was unaffected throughout. The researchers concluded that the increase in plasma norepinephrine was due to the decline in glucose and was a marker of biological changes upon the initiation of starvation.

Given the increase in energy expenditure, this was an indication that the metabolic rate had increased.

Aside from these benefits, there is also evidence that IF increases the secretion of HGH, or human growth hormone, which helps in muscle building and fat loss, as well as reduces the levels of insulin in the body which makes the fat more accessible to burn (Gunnars, 2017).

Following intermittent fasting, the plan is quite straight forward. There aren't many rules or regulations for you to follow, unlike other diets. However, there are some mental blocks that always trip people up.

So let me first address these bogus claims, and then I'll show you the different methods by which you can implement IF in your life.

### *Pattern*

Let me say this right off the bat: human beings are perfectly capable of functioning without food for long periods of time (Gunnars, 2017). I'm not talking a few hours; I'm talking days. In ancient times, it was common for our ancestors to go without food for days. After all, it's not as if deer and other food simply offered themselves up to be eaten willingly.

Thus, if you're worried about failing to function or concerned about your activity levels dropping, rest assured. Your concerns are legitimate, but your brain is amplifying the doubt within because you're so used to a particular pattern of eating that anything else strikes you as being unnatural. Never mind the fact that fasting from time to time is the natural way to eat, as opposed to eating three to four times per day (Gunnars, 2017).

In other words, you've formed a habit and habits take time to change. IF's pattern is something that models the body's natural activity pattern. It calls for periods of fasting broken up by periods of eating, done in cycles. The most significant advantage IF provides is that it doesn't provide you with a list of foods to avoid or eat.

Instead, you only need to eat according to your fasting and feeding pattern, and the rest takes care of itself! There are multiple ways to practice intermittent fasting, so let's take a quick look at these.

### 16/8 Method

This method is also referred to as the "leangains protocol," which was developed by Swedish nutritionist Martin Berkhan. Leangains is probably the most effective IF protocol out there and reached the peak of its popularity around 2014. Unfortunately, this is when the mainstream fitness industry got wind of it, and all sorts of wrong and frankly idiotic information were peddled.

At its core, leangains are all about eating your meals within an eight-hour window and fasting for sixteen hours. Berkhan recommends adding your sleep periods to your fasting times, so if you sleep for eight hours per day, you'll be eating for eight hours, sleeping for eight and fasting awake for eight hours. It is this third period that can seem challenging.

Given this sort of a breakup, you will have to skip one of the traditionally accepted meals in society. Berkhan recommends skipping breakfast, which will probably ring alarm bells of all kinds within your head, but is the most effective way of implementing leangains (Berkhan, 2015). The method does take some getting used to and goes well beyond eating for eight and fasting for sixteen hours. You will need to train heavy as well as cycle your eating pattern based on whether you're working out that day or not. Doing this can seem a bit overwhelming, so let's take a closer look.

## *A Deeper Look at 16/8*

There are no guidelines as to which time of the day you need to remain fasted or fed - this is entirely up to you. Losing fat is ultimately a question of how many calories you eat. As long as you eat less than you burn, you'll lose weight and gain more definition. Now, having said that, this doesn't mean you can eat whatever you want. Yes, technically, even if you do eat chocolate cake all day, and in amounts that provide less energy than what you need, you will lose weight.

However, weight loss is very different from fat loss. When losing weight, you can lose muscle as well, which is not what you want to be doing. So, yeah, sorry to say, your chocolate cake diet ain't gonna work! That doesn't mean you need to place yourself in food purgatory. Since you're fasting for as long as you are, you can get away with eating a bit more unhealthy stuff than usual. Obviously, this is not recommended, but my point is don't be worried about missing out.

Berkhan recommends three protocols based on when you choose to workout (Berkhan, 2015). And yes, you will need to work out hard and heavy. A lot of us girls have been brainwashed into thinking that if we lift heavy weights, we'll end up looking like one of those Mr. Olympia types. Another example of the utter nonsense that gets peddled. If you train like a man does, you'll look like a goddess. There, I said it.

Not because of some male-specific training regimen; it's just that when you workout with heavier loads, you're forcing your body to become stronger and put on more muscle and lose fat. In turn, this helps you look and feel younger, and you will also have more strength. Unless you choose to take steroids or hormones of any kind, you will never lose your feminine shape and body, so don't worry about that.

You can workout fasted, after one meal, or after two meals. There is no fixed number of meals you need to eat within the feeding phase. Those that workout after one meal will usually find it easier to eat just a meal with a small snack. Those who have more normal working schedules will find that working out after two meals is easier, with one meal post workout.

## *Meal Breakdown*

With leangains, your most substantial meal should be consumed after your workout. The largest meal is defined as the one which has over 60% of your required calories. Now, word of warning, you will need to calculate your macros - that is the amount of fat, carbs, and protein you will need to eat depending on your goals with the diet (Berkhan, 2015).

The best way to do this is to use the macro calculator on Berkhan's website and calculate how much you need to eat to reach your goals. If you are overweight for your height and age, you will need to eat less than 'maintenance,' which is the number of calories you will need to eat to remain at the same weight.

Choosing to train fasted early in the morning is the fastest way to lose fat as soon as possible. However, this is also the toughest, since it calls for enormous mental strength. You will also need to supplement your diet with a lot of BCAA, which is a supplement I will cover later in the book. To be frank, fasted training gave me a lot of gains, but it was just too difficult and exhausting to implement.

The next option you have is to train after one meal. So if your eating window is between 12PM-8PM, which is what most people normally choose, you could eat your first meal, which is around 30% of the calories you need at 12 PM and then workout at 2 PM. Berkhan recommends working out no more than a couple of hours after finishing your meal.

Your post workout meal, which should be eaten within an hour of finishing your workout, can be had around 4-5PM, and this will be 60% of your calories. The remaining 10% can be eaten around 7:30 PM to finish off your feeding phase.

The last option is to workout after two meals. In this scenario, you will eat at 12 PM, then have your snack around 4-5PM or right before you get off work, and then workout after that. Your last meal, which will be the biggest meal of the day, will be post workout, and you end your feeding phase with this.

Personally, the final option of working out after two meals was what worked wonders for me. It was effortless to implement with my work schedule and other things going on. Again, you can adjust your feeding/fasting window to any time of the day to help make it easier to implement. Just don't break it up into multiple windows, which won't give you the same metabolic effect.

### Workouts

Berkhan calls for heavy, full body exercises such as squats, deadlifts, bench presses, and overhead presses for maximum gain (Berkhan, 2015). These workouts will build your strength and combined with the diet regimen; it will melt the fat right off you. The biggest challenge you will find, as a woman, is doing this in a gym.

You will encounter stares from the other gym goers when they see a girl lifting heavy weights and hanging around the big dude area of the gym floor. You will feel self-conscious, but here's a secret: Those big guys staring at you are actually admiring you. The stereotype of the gym rat who goes around laughing at people is just that. More often than not, you'll find that those gym bros will walk over and give you some tips. It's their way of showing you respect.

So don't be afraid of going in there and doing what you need to do! For more in-depth and scientifically researched articles on this topic, make sure to check our Berkhan's website, https://leangains.com/. His writing style will take some getting used to, but ultimately, his website is extremely informative.

### *Drawbacks of 16/8*

Leangains is a tough regimen to follow. While the macro calculation is pretty simple, the real test comes when you're two or three weeks into the program, and your lifts start getting heavy. There is also a temptation to complicate the program as well, and Berkhan's writing doesn't help in this regard.

While his focus is primarily on his clients, he does give a lot of information for free on his website. However, a lot of it is filled with deep scientific jargon, and he doesn't make it easy to understand what he's conveying, leaving it up to you to do further research and go down a nutritional rabbit hole.

Thus, if you hit a plateau or any difficulty, you will not find too much-personalized information. Over and above this, if you're not used to working out in a gym and have never done this before, you will find leangains and Berkhan's general tough love approach to things a bit too much to stomach.

This method is perhaps suited for those who already have some experience with IF and exercising as opposed to those who are doing this for the first time. If you're one of the latter, this will be one of those sink or swim type of situations, and it can get deeply uncomfortable at times. There are alternative approaches to IF, however, as we'll now see.

### Eat Stop Eat

This program was also designed by a nutritionist, Brad Pilon, who implements IF in a different manner from how Berkhan does. Instead of fasting every single day, Pilon recommends fasting entirely at least once and up to twice per week, while regularly eating on the remaining days ("Eat Stop Eat Review (2019): A Legit Diet For Weight Loss? Or Fake Fad?", 2019).

You can choose to calculate your maintenance calorie rate with this, which will make your life easier. If not, you will need to track your weight and adjust accordingly. Either way, this is not as difficult as it sounds, and you shouldn't let this scare you away.

The underlying logic behind eat stop eat is to create a caloric deficit which will help you lose fat in a healthy manner. Traditional methods of losing fat involve a lot of macro calculation and maintenance, which a majority of dieters don't have the mental energy or willingness to do.

By prescribing up to two days of fasting per week, Pilon takes this issue out of the equation in a precise manner. Let's look at how this works in depth.

### A Deeper Look at Eat Stop Eat

Pilon recommends women eat two thousand calories per day and men eat around two thousand five hundred per day during their feeding days ("Eat Stop Eat Review (2019): A Legit Diet For Weight Loss? Or Fake Fad?", 2019). The number of fasting days per week should be at least one and a maximum of two. If you choose to fast two days per week, make sure they are not consecutive days.

When your body is in a fasted state, it will turn to any and all nutrition sources within. Thus, fat becomes a source of nutrition and will be burned as fuel. Not to mention, the fasting days give your body to the chance to cleanse itself and get rid of any unwanted toxins within it ("Eat Stop Eat Review (2019): A Legit Diet For Weight Loss? Or Fake Fad?", 2019).

The fasted state does pose a few challenges, though. Your body is liable to interpret the fasting period as being an unnatural one and is likely to start loading up on fat instead of burning it. Because fat is your body's emergency reserve for energy. Thus, your muscles will be burned in an effort to maintain your fat. The way to avoid this is to work out intensely during your feeding days.

By working out, you increase your muscle mass and communicate that this muscle should be preserved. Thus, when you fast, the body gets the message that the fasting phase is planned and that nutrition will arrive soon. After all, you wouldn't be exerting yourself hard if there was a famine going on, would you?

Thus, via the two fasting days, you end up creating a caloric deficit, up to 10% according to Pilon ("Eat Stop Eat Review (2019): A Legit Diet For Weight Loss? Or Fake Fad?", 2019), and you will lose fat. He doesn't provide any specific guidelines for what to eat and leaves it up to you to decide, as long as you hit the recommended two thousand calorie number (for a woman).

The time you wish to start your fast doesn't matter. For example, you could eat a meal at 8:30 PM and then continue your fast until 8:30 PM the following day. From a practical perspective, timing this is tough. After all, you need to nourish yourself once your fast is broken. The best way to achieve this is to start your fasting period in the afternoon and have it end on the following afternoon. This way, you've given yourself enough time to consume the required number of calories for that day.

## *Workouts*

It is best to avoid workouts on your fasted days since you'll only be consuming water or low-calorie drinks like sparkling water. During your feeding days, it is best to perform strength training exercises, although Pilon doesn't call for as intense a workout routine as with leangains.

He does, however, prioritize strength building over cardio. Cardio is generally used to lose fat, but with your diet taking care of that already, performing only cardio will cause you to lose muscle. Thus, focus on training for strength and performing exercises in the 6-12 rep range.

If you don't know what a rep is or are wondering what exercises you should perform, don't worry, I'll cover all of this in a later chapter. For now, remember that you ought to focus on strength training and not just cardio.

You can exercise three to four days per week and follow one of the recommended workout programs which I've listed later in this book.

## *Drawbacks of Eat Stop Eat*

While providing a more straightforward template to follow, Eat Stop Eat is more challenging to put into practice at the end of the day. The biggest reason for this is the constant weight tracking you need to do and the possibility of overeating when you come out of your fast.

The fasting period is far more drastic as compared to leangains, and this will tempt a lot of people to overeat. Not to mention, the difficulty of tracking calories before and after you break your fast. The method is a bit unclear about this, and Pilon seems to suggest that the calories will even out over time, thanks to the deficit building up.

Since this is an IF method, there is no specific nutritional guide, and the primary source of information is Pilon's book, *Eat Stop Eat*. Overall, this is a very effective method if you can manage to implement it, and the results it provides are very real. By relying on basic IF principles, and by delivering a simple template, the method is well worth a shot.

## 5:2

The last intermittent fasting protocol is the most beginner friendly and is the easiest to follow and understand. Title 5:2, the diet calls for eating what you want for five days of the week and on two days, eating just five hundred calories. The intention is to create a caloric deficit via the two fasting days, which are supposed to be non-consecutive (Bjarnadottir, 2018).

There are no other calorie restrictions with this diet, and it is essentially a simplification of the previous two methods. Eat Stop Eat has become the most popular type of intermittent fasting protocol right now, and the reason for this is the minimal change that is required to implement it.

By not having to calculate a lot of macros or even calories, you're free to eat as you've been doing this far. It kicks in only on the two days you have to fast and restrict yourself to five hundred calories. Over and above this, you can follow your chosen regimen of exercise, which will boost your fat loss as well (Bjarnadottir, 2018).

That's pretty much all there is to it, really! I don't even need an in-depth section to explain this further. There are, however, some cons of this method you need to be aware of.

## *Drawbacks of 5:2*

Now, I mean this in the nicest way possible, but you must understand that this method is a hack. It will work for those who have a lot of weight to lose. Once you lose that excess weight, though, you will hit a plateau since the regimen isn't very structured.

The reason most people gain weight is that they don't know how to structure their diets. By removing this requirement, 5:2 writes a great elevator pitch for itself, but it falls short in the long run. Here's the thing: While sticking to a diet regimen is detail oriented and painful, it exists for a reason. You must put in the work to see the results.

Personally, I think the 5:2 seems to market itself as the method that takes out that complexity and appeals to our lazier sides. So you will see results at first, but don't expect it to work out over the long term. Its lack of any complexity is what causes it to fail.

So thus far, we've seen three IF methods with one being a bit complex, another being a little less and one having no complexity at all. Complexity is no guarantee of effectiveness, but neither is a complete lack of it. Ultimately, you need to look at which method you can implement the best in your life.

From a results standpoint, over the long term, there is no doubt that leangains provides the best results (Gunnars, 2017). The method not only cuts fat but also helps your body remain leaner for longer since it adjusts to the new regimen. The first mental block, with regards to skipping a meal, usually breakfast, requires energy to deal with, but this is repaid many times over.

Now if this were simply a book on intermittent fasting, I'd send you on your way with these words. However, the problems soon became real to me since implementing all of this is not an easy task. Now, this is where the ketogenic diet takes out all guesswork. By implementing a definite diet plan which you can follow, you boost the effectiveness of IF.

Why don't the creators of the previous IF plans do this, you might be wondering? Well, Berkhan does provide macro nutrition guidelines on his website, and even Pilon recommends a certain macro ratio. However, they don't insist on it, because they expect the people following it to use some common sense, according to them, and figure it out.

However, I aim to remove all the guesswork for you and give you a definite guide. I'm going to spend some time now talking about the ketogenic diet and how you can successfully implement it in your life.

## KETOGENIC DIET

The ketogenic diet has been prescribed as a method of managing both diabetes and for those suffering from seizures since the 1930s (Kubala, 2018). The diet is also known by its other moniker, LCHF, which stands for low carb, high fat. In a nutshell, this pretty much explains what Keto is all about.

The diet calls for reducing all forms of carbs down to the bare minimum and in its place, eating fat with a decent amount of protein. The keto diet has several benefits and can help with health issues ranging from obesity to diabetes. Several studies have been conducted that prove beyond a shadow of a doubt the efficacy of this diet. Here's just a small sample:

Obesity: A study conducted in 2003 placed sixty-four subjects into two groups and divided them based on their diet. One was placed on a high-fat diet, while the other was on a high carb, low-fat diet (Foster et al., 2003).

The researchers found that the group on the low carb diet lost significantly more weight than the other group, which was on a regular diet. This effect was observed at both the three and six-month mark.

In this study, the rate of attrition was high, and thus, it was not as effective over twelve months. However, at the six-month mark, there was no doubt as to which was more effective in tackling obesity.

Diabetes: In a study in 2006, Type 2 diabetes patients were randomly grouped into two groups, again differentiated based on their diets. One was on a low-fat diet while the other was on a high-fat diet.

Here's what the researchers concluded (Daly et al., 2006):

*Fat loss was greater in the low-carbohydrate (LC) group (−3.55 ± 0.63, mean ± sem) vs. −0.92 ± 0.40 kg, P = 0.001) and cholesterol :*

*high-density lipoprotein (HDL) ratio improved (−0.48 ± 0.11 vs. −0.10 ± 0.10, P = 0.01).*

*However, relatively saturated fat intake was higher (13.9 ± 0.71 vs. 11.0 ± 0.47% of dietary intake, P < 0.001), although total intakes were moderate.*

As you can see, along with the weight loss, levels of HDL, or good cholesterol, also improved. This study confirms why the keto diet is recommended as a means of managing Type 2 diabetes in patients.

Brain Cancer: While the keto diet is not a cure for this malignant disease, researchers observed a remarkable reduction in tumor sizes in patients. A study performed in 2007 (Zhou et al., 2007) found that tumor sizes decreased by 65% and 35% respectively, and this enhanced the survival rate as compared to the group which was on the standard diet.

Aside from this, glucose levels dropped and, as expected, ketone levels increased. The density of the tumors was far smaller as compared to the group on the regular high carb diet. The researchers postulated that the smaller tumor size could be explained by the fact that the tumors could not metabolize ketones for energy and hence shrunk.

These studies are just meant to show you how effective the keto diet is. To understand why and how this works, we need to understand an important concept: ketosis.

### *Ketosis*

Ketosis refers to when the body starts burning fat for fuel instead of glucose. Let me back up for a second and explain the body's relationship to glucose and carbs. The body's first option for burning fuel to power you is glucose. Glucose is a sugar that is derived from burning carbs.

Thus, whenever you eat something, it is the carbs that get burned first, as a priority, and then if there's any more need for fuel, the body moves onto fat and then protein, which is just your muscles. If you remove the primary source of fuel, the body will be forced to move onto burning fat for fuel. Thus, the fat that you have stored in your body gets burned, and this is why eating fat makes you lose fat. Yes, I understand how convoluted that sentence is.

Your body doesn't just snap into a fat burning mode, though. For most of us, it is used to burning carbs, and thus when the supply is cut off, the body goes into a twilight zone sort of mode, where it doesn't know what is going on. During this time, it will not burn your fat efficiently, and when it finally gets the message that no more carbs are forthcoming, it switches over to burning fat.

The burning of fat releases a fatty acid that contains molecules called ketones. Ketones can be detected in your blood and urine, and their production is what is referred to as a state of ketosis. The objective of the Keto diet is to keep you in ketosis for as long as possible.

Eating too many carbs will throw you out of ketosis since your body will start burning glucose instead. Thus, keeping your carbs as low as possible is vital. Could you eliminate carbs completely? Sure, you could. However, the energy it takes to remove them entirely doesn't provide as much return for your time as simply minimizing them.

## *Keto Food*

Keto emphasizes food high in protein and fat, preferably both. This means the below foods are perfectly acceptable on this diet:

- Meat (preferably lean)

- Fatty Fish

- Chicken (lean or fatty cut)

- Bacon

- Low carb veggies like lettuce, spinach, broccoli

- Eggs

- Butter

- Cheese

- Cream

- Olive oil, Seed Oil

- Nuts and Seeds

- Tofu

- Tempeh, Seitan

- The foods to avoid are the following:

- Grains

- Legumes

- Starchy Vegetables like carrots, potatoes

- Fruits

- Beans

- Sugary foods and drink

- Bread

- Pasta

- Flour products

Keto usually presents a problem for those who are used to consuming a lot of bread or flour-based products such as pasta. For most Americans, in other words, it is quite a change that requires planning. However, with the right preparation, which I will show you, you can easily implement this in your life.

Another point to note is that while red meat is perfectly fine on this diet, it is still wise to minimize it and stick to the leaner cuts, red meat contains a lot of saturated fat. Saturated fat is a tricky beast on which there isn't a lot of conclusive research.

Here's what we know: Excess levels of saturated fat cause cancer and other malignant diseases (Gunnars, 2017). However, some degree of saturated fat is required to possess good health. Thus, the best we can say at this point is to simply minimize it, but don't eliminate it. Practically speaking, this would mean eating red meat once or maybe twice per week, relying on chicken, turkey, and fish to make up the content of your meals.

Another sticking point is the lack of fruits on the diet. Fruits contain naturally occurring sugars, which are perfectly healthy but will throw you out of ketosis and so are not allowed. Make sure you eat a lot of green leafy vegetables, and you'll get all the micronutrients and vitamins you need.

### Types of Keto Diets

While the standard keto diet, or SKD, is the one which is most widely followed. Some variations serve their own purposes. For your purposes, the SKD will be more than enough, but it's still worthwhile to look at the variations in case one of them makes sense to you.

SKD or Standard Keto Diet: This is the regular diet wherein you consume around 80-100g of protein per day and keep your carbs below 30g per day. The remainder of your calories come from fat. As you can see, this entails calculating your calories, but because you'll be combining your keto diet with IF, don't worry about hitting your calorie targets or whether you should eat something or not.

What you should do, however, is get a rough idea of how much food makes up your calorie quota for the day.

HPKD- The High Protein Keto Diet is aimed at those who wish to gain muscle with cutting fat as a secondary concern. In this regimen, the amount of protein is increased to almost one gram per pound of body weight, and carbs are maintained below thirty grams. The rest of the calories are gained from fat.

CKD and TKD - The cyclical and targeted ketogenic diets are meant for those who go through extremely intense and heavy workouts. Working out and lifting weight requires the body's anaerobic facility to be high, and the keto diet tends to suppress this. Thus, with these diets, you load on carbs before working out and then aim to return to ketosis as soon as possible, post workout.

For you, the SKD combined with IF will more than do the job, as it did for me. The variations of keto are mostly for people who are very experienced and have demanding workout routines, and you ought not to worry about any of that.

Given the benefits, combining them seems like a no brainer. However, you might be worried about inheriting the difficulties of both as well.

Well, fear not, this is why I've created the next chapter, which will give you a thirty-day plan to prep for the changes you're about to make. This next chapter will help you transition into this new regimen, and all you have to do is follow it.

# CHAPTER 2:

# THIRTY DAY KETO PREP GUIDE

# (FAMILY FRIENDLY)

So now that you know what IF and keto are about separately, it's time to put these together into a framework that you can use to lose fat quickly and in a healthy manner. The basic structure is simple enough: you need to follow an intermittent fasting protocol and eat only the foods which are permitted on the ketogenic diet. Easy peasy, right?

Well, it is as simple as that! However, a lot of people fail at this simply because they take it easy and don't prepare. If you fail to prepare, you prepare to fail! I'm not sure who said that originally, but I once heard Usain Bolt say it, and I'm willing to take his word for it.

In this chapter, I'm going to talk all about prep work. The good news is from an IF perspective; there isn't much you need to do. Keto deserves a good look, however, since you're probably not used to eating this way.

So, let's jump in!

## INTERMITTENT FASTING PREP

The first thing you need to do is to decide which protocol you wish to follow. The previous chapter gave you three to choose from, the 16/8, Eat Stop Eat, and 5:2. I'm a huge fan of the 16/8, which is the leangains technique.

Not to say that the other two are ineffective. It comes down to your personal choice. However, if you're one of those people who is sick of research and want something cut and dried, read on!

### *My Recommended IF Protocol*

There are no surprises here - I recommend 16/8 all the way. If you are serious about it and are comfortable with digesting the lengthy nutritional treatises Berkhan writes about on his blog, I'd say go for the full leangains approach, which involves cycling your macros on your rest days. If this puts you off, don't worry. There's a simple solution.

Don't worry about cycling carbs or even working out heavy and hard as he recommends. Instead, focus on eating for eight hours and fasting for sixteen. Work out as hard as you can for as long as you can. Now, this doesn't mean you should jog in place for fifteen minutes and call it quits.

Instead, be sincere about it and definitely do some form of strength training. I've laid out a beginner strength conditioning plan for you in a later chapter, so don't worry about having to research it all by yourself. Keep it simple in terms of this protocol. Which means you don't have to worry about cycling your macros or anything of that sort.

You'll be following the keto diet anyway, so it shouldn't be much of a concern to you. Here's the important bit though: you should define your goal before you begin. Sure, your goal is to lose fat and so on and so forth. However, it is best to write down the reason you want to lose fat in the first place.

Do you want to have a sexy body? Sure! But why? What does this give you? You see, I'm trying to ask you to reflect on the real emotional reason you want to do this. Everybody has their own reasons for pursuing things in their life, and the more you are in touch with the real reason, the better you'll push yourself through the pain period.

Make no mistake, IF combined with keto, takes work. It's my job to prepare you for what lies ahead, and I'm not going to sugarcoat it for you. To be able to make it to the other side and condition your mind and body, you need a really good reason which will push you through and get you off your backside, up and running.

Once you have your reasons down, it's time to fix your fasting and feeding intervals. The interval that works for most people is to eat between 12-12:30 PM and 8-8:30 PM. Assuming you go to bed at 10 PM and wake up at 6 AM, this means you will be skipping breakfast.

If you don't wish to skip breakfast, you'll be skipping dinner. Neither of these options is socially too friendly, but given that people usually don't meet each other over breakfast, it is socially more palatable to skip breakfast. If you have a family, this will take some explaining, but be firm and stick to your resolutions.

I'll talk about this in more detail, but you really want to recruit some additional help for the first week. If you have a spouse or significant other and if the two of you have kids, then you will definitely need help. This is because your body has been conditioned to eat soon after waking up, and during the first week, it will scream in protest at the new order of things. Keto brings its challenges, so be prepared and get some help.

If you live alone, you probably won't need additional help, and it's nothing you cannot manage. It's just that kids and a family need extra attention, which is why I recommended it. The best time to implement the new IF plus keto regimen is over the weekend. If done right, by the time Monday rolls around you'll have adjusted to the keto and your morning hunger pangs will have significantly subsided. You'll also have gotten rid of your crankiness over the weekend.

So once you've circled the date, it's time to calculate your macros! As recommended in the previous chapter, use the calculator on Berkhan's website or simply Google "leangains macro calculator." Remember, you will need to be in a caloric deficit since your goal is to lose weight. In other words, you will be eating less than what you need to maintain your current weight.

Now here's the tricky bit. Every calculator out there requires an input with regards to your activity level. The levels range from sedentary to extremely active. For the most part, you will fall between sedentary to moderately active. Unless you're a pro athlete of some sort (in which case you don't need this book) or work in construction all day long, you're not going to be highly active.

A good rule of thumb is to estimate what you think your activity level is, and then choose the level below it. This way, you're playing it safe and won't need to change things down the road. Once you input all your numbers, that's it! You will receive a number that represents your daily maintenance number.

This number represents how many calories you need to eat in order to maintain your current weight. Since you want to lose weight, subtract 25% from this number (in other words, calculate 75% of this number), and that is the number of calories you need to eat every day, within your eight-hour window.

Plan to have at least three meals. If you're not comfortable eating large meals or embarrassed by it, which is a common girl problem, then break it down into smaller meals and eat every couple hours or so. Remember to eat 60% of your calories after your workout.

### *When Should I Work Out?*

Work out whenever you damn well, please. As much as possible, avoid working out fasted. I know I said this is the quickest way to lose fat in the previous chapter, but you'll recall I also said it's mentally exhausting. Try playing around with this once you've built up some experience. For now, make sure you work out only after eating your first meal, at the very least.

If you're used to getting up in the morning to go jogging, I'd advise shelving those plans for now. Try to reschedule your workout for another time of the day. A lot of the time, I've noticed women will do anything to avoid going to the gym for fear of being laughed at. I'm telling you, once again, that there's nothing to be afraid of. So be brave and do this!

From an IF perspective, this is really all you need to prep for. The keto side of things requires more work, but don't worry. It's nothing you can't handle!

## KETO PREP

Keto prep mostly involves getting your kitchen in order and stocking up on the right stuff in your home. In short, make it as easy as you can for you to follow the diet and do not give your brain any excuses to duck out of this. You'll be surprised at how much of a genius your brain can be when it comes to shirking responsibilities.

Let's take this step by step and being with your pots and pans.

### *Utensils and Kitchen Equipment*

If you want to make life easy for yourself, get yourself an oven. More than anything else, it is the oven which will save you a ton of time and headache over what to cook and what not to. Most homes come equipped with one these days and if not, consider buying an external one. I'm not talking about those microwave/oven/grill posers, but the real things.

Next, get yourself some baking pans and ramekins. Ramekins are those little cups you bake with in order to make small pies and tarts. You'll be breaking a lot of eggs into these bad boys, so get yourself some good quality ones. You don't need too many baking pans - a medium and a large one will do. See if you can get a bread pan and double that as a baking dish. This will become clear in the next chapter, so trust me on this one.

The next two pieces of kitchen equipment you ought to have are a skillet and a grill. A grill is optional, but it gives a nice change of pace to things. A grill is also a handy substitute for an oven, although it doesn't have the same versatility. If you don't want an oven or think you can't afford one, go for a simple grill. It doesn't need to be one of those tailgating monstrosities, just a simple one. A skillet is a must have, since it'll make your life a whole lot easier.

Presumably, you already have a kitchen knife and forks, or if you're particularly adventurous, a spork (or fpoon), so I'm not going to go too much into that.

### *But I Hate Cooking!*

Some of us love to cook, and some hate it. Well, for those who love to cook, this shouldn't pose too much of a challenge. If you are less than enthusiastic, though, you're going to have to suck it up. Also, cooking a decent meal isn't as hard as you think. After all, you're not presenting your dish for the privilege of being yelled at by Gordon Ramsay.

It's just you eating your cooking, so deal! Besides, I've outlined a full cooking game plan for you in the next chapter, which will make your life easier. Don't worry; your meals will taste delicious. It will require you to put just a little time in the kitchen and won't involve anything extraordinarily difficult.

If you don't know how to cook, well, this is the best time to learn how to boil an egg! Seriously though, if you don't know how to cook, master some basic cooking skills first and practice for a week or two before starting. You'll only sabotage yourself through a lack of preparation otherwise.

If you have a full-time job, then no matter what, you need to plan on packing your meals with you on the go. The great thing about the keto diet is that salads are ubiquitous, so you'll be spoiled for choice in this regard. A large number of keto meals boil down to grilling or baking some meat, throwing in on top of a salad and munching that. Throw some eggs or avocado on top of it to give it some variety.

Also, you'll be pleased to know that lasagna is entirely keto, so you won't have to stay away from Italian goodness if you're a fan of that cuisine. Plus, you can now totally indulge in the cheese platter after dinner. Dessert also opens up new avenues in the form of dark chocolate, and once you've eaten this, you'll wonder why you ever liked milk chocolate.

Oh yeah, whipped cream and creams of all sorts are OK now, so there's that. All in all, don't worry. There are a ton of meal choices for you to indulge in!

## *The Fog*

We've now come to the biggest hurdle you'll need to overcome when adopting the keto diet. Termed variously as the fog or the keto haze and so on, this is a mental state that everyone experiences upon first beginning the diet. To understand why and how this happens, we need to step back a bit into the basics covered in the previous chapter.

You will recall that the keto diet works wonders thanks to a process called ketosis, which is when your body begins to burn fat as fuel instead of its preferred source, glucose. When you first start the keto diet, your body is still accustomed to burning and receiving carbs as the major source of nutrition.

Our bodies are remarkably engineered to help us survive many conditions. For every scenario, the body has a backup of some sort to help us deal and survive. When you first starve your body of carbs, it simply turns inward and starts burning up the existing stores of glucose, reasoning that more will be on its way shortly and that there's no need to panic.

Once these existing stores are burned off, the body lies in wait for more carbs to enter the system. Soon, it begins to realize that no more is forthcoming and that it needs to activate plan B. Plan B is burning the fat stores within the body and prioritizing the burning of fat since no carbs or minimal carbs are forthcoming.

Our bodies take around three to four days, at the most a week, to change over and adjust to the new regimen. During this period, your body is not yet accustomed to burning fat in the most efficient manner possible, and thus, whatever is being burned isn't providing the greatest amount of energy it can.

Thus, you will feel a significant drop in energy and will feel weaker. Mind you; this is just a feeling associated with a lack of energy. You aren't growing weak. You will experience irritation at the slightest things simply because you don't have the energy to deal with them.

For some people, the fog doesn't really ever go away because their bodies are not physically suited to the keto diet. If this happens to you, you should consult your doctor. For the rest of us, the fog subsides within a week at the most, with a couple of days being the usual fog period.

The best way to beat the fog is to decrease your consumption of carbs drastically. On average, in America, we consume around 400g of carbs per day. By cutting this to less than 30g, you will force your body into ketosis faster only because it has to; otherwise, it will starve.

It is recommended that you implement the keto diet over a weekend since you don't have to deal with your office colleagues or traffic and all the attendant nonsense it brings. If you are a stay at home mom, though, a weekday is your best bet since you'll have the house to yourself and can carry things out in peace.

Ultimately, figure out what will work best in your life and do that.

## *Shopping*

This is the easy bit. Load up on the keto staples below:

- Eggs
- Lean meat like beef and chicken
- Frozen shrimp
- Green vegetables
- Butter
- Dark Chocolate
- Low carb veggies like broccoli and cauliflower
- Avocado

- Canned tuna, sardines, and mackerel

- Mayonnaise (natural and full fat)

- Mozzarella, Parmesan, and Ricotta cheese

- Olive or nut oil like coconut, almond, etc.

- Coconut flour

- Spices

You could also opt for indulgences like the following:

- Salmon

- Fresh Tuna cuts

- Fresh Crab and Shellfish

That is all there is to shop for the keto diet. From these base ingredients, you will be able to create a wide variety of delicious dishes.

If budget is an issue, reduce your shopping staples to the following:

- Chicken breasts and thighs

- Mozzarella cheese

- Spinach and lettuce

- Mayonnaise

- Canned tuna

- Coconut oil

- Spices - spice mix, five spice mix, pepper, etc.

## *Restaurants*

Not everyone can always eat at home all the time. It's great to go out and treat yourself. When eating out, due to the restrictions of the keto diet, you will find it difficult to dine out at ethnic restaurants that favor rice or a substitute and bread of some kind. To deal with this, you have two options.

Either you don't eat this type of food, or you make a meal here part of your cheat meal. A cheat meal is a release valve of sorts where you can allow yourself to break your diet rules. A cheat meal doesn't give you the luxury of eating how much ever you want. You can break your rules but in moderation. For example, if you want pizza, then instead of eating an entire pie, have a slice. Instead of a huge sundae, have a scoop of your favorite ice cream.

When ordering at a restaurant, stick to meat and salads, since that's pretty much what the keto diet prescribes. You can enjoy a cheesecake dessert as long as you minimize the crumble and keep in mind the number of calories present. A cheat meal doesn't give you the luxury of blowing your calorie counts out of the water. Feel free to not eat to a deficit, but don't overdo it.

# THE NEXT 30 DAYS

So, having finished prepping and mentally prepared yourself for the upcoming challenge, let's look at what you can expect for the next four weeks. Use this as a guide to check in and evaluate whether or not you're on the right path.

Don't expect to get everything right the first time. Everyone makes mistakes - there's no other way to learn. What matters is how you work to rectify it.

### *Week One*

This will be your most challenging week. Hopefully, you've prepared for this as detailed in the previous sections and planned your meals out in advance. Also, be prepared for the keto fog and get ready for some low energy moments and general irritability.

It is a good idea to skip any workouts for the first few days until you've adjusted to the fog. Also, remember that your feeding window isn't something that needs to end on the dot at eight hours. If you go over by ten or fifteen minutes, this is fine. Your body doesn't measure time in such terms, so don't be a perfectionist about it.

This week is all about tracking, which is something I'll talk about in a later chapter. For now, remember to keep tracking your metrics as mentioned, and keep your carbs low.

You will feel massive cravings for bread or wheat products, and this can be a challenge to overcome. Over and above, this will be your cravings for breakfast. With the latter, you can drink some water or coffee without sugar or sweeteners of any kind to help tide you over. If it becomes a bit too much, consider sleeping later so that you don't face too much of a fasting window when you wake up.

As far as the craving for bread goes, one of the best ways to overcome this is to eat something crunchy like lettuce. Lettuce has trace amounts of carbs, and simply chewing on this will keep your mouth occupied and your brain will quiet down. The key is to keep chewing something and not eating if you know what I mean.

Generally, by the fifth day, your fog should have disappeared entirely if it hasn't, talk to your doctor and see what they suggest. For some people, it can last as long as a week. In extremely rare cases it takes up to two weeks.

If you're not feeling a fog, then there are two possible things happening. One, your body has perfectly adjusted to the new diet, so congratulations! The second scenario is that you're eating more carbs than you imagined. Track whether your body is in ketosis (I'll cover this in the tracking chapter) and check to see if this is true if your test results are positive then great! Keep doing what you're doing.

## Week Two

You should have started working out by now, and you will have certainly lost weight by this point. Note I said weight, not fat. Once you stop eating carbs, your body doesn't need to store as much water within, and this is flushed out. So expect to pee a lot more during the middle of the first week through this week.

If you are still experiencing the fog, then see your doctor. Perhaps the diet isn't for you. By this point, you should be comfortable with your fasting and feeding windows and given that you're now working out, you will begin to feel hunger pangs at night or in the morning when you skip a meal.

These are extremely challenging to deal with, and you can adopt coping strategies like drinking water or unsweetened coffee to minimize this. Keep referring back to your reason to do this and keep reminding yourself of what it is you wish to achieve by following your diet.

Keep enforcing your discipline, and it will become a muscle.

## Week Three

If you've been maintaining a healthy deficit, you should be losing, at most, a pound and a half per week. So by the end of this week, you should have lost four to five pounds max. If you've lost less than this, don't worry, a pound or even half a pound per week is perfectly healthy.

If you haven't lost any weight or have put on weight, then your macro calculations are wrong, and you need to recalculate. Again, this is covered in detail in the tracking chapter.

Your calorie deficit is building up now, and your hunger pangs will be huge. This week is a turning point of sorts, where your hunger pains become more prominent than usual, but your mental ability to deal with them is also strong.

Stick to your discipline for this week, and soon, you'll be able to handle your hunger really well. It will never really go away, but you'll be able to rationalize it by thinking of hunger as fat being burned within you.

### Week Four

By the end of this week, you should ideally have lost anywhere from two to six pounds of fat. If you've maintained a caloric deficit of 25% throughout, then you should expect to lose around four pounds. If you've lost more than this, then it's not just fat that has been lost, but muscle. So, recalculate your macros and start eating a bit more and keep tracking things as described in the tracking chapter.

So, there you have it! A simple four-week plan to get you losing fat in a healthy manner while gaining strength. Remember to prepare well and follow the steps outlined, and you'll be just fine.

Now, a question that usually arises is what is one supposed to eat when breaking your fast. Are there any dietary guidelines? How about cheat meals, and what's the deal with them? Well, this is what I'll cover next.

# CHAPTER 3:

# WHAT THE HECK DO YOU EAT
# WHEN BREAKING YOUR FAST?

The breaking of your fast is a crucial moment since your first meal usually sets the tone for how well you'll be able to adhere to your rules. Most people approach this meal with a pang of ravenous hunger, understandably so, and tend to gorge themselves. It is tempting to make this the biggest meal of your day, but the reality is that you need to determine the size of this meal based on your routine.

In this chapter, I'll lay out everything you need to take into consideration when breaking your fast and in designing your meals.

# WHAT TO EAT AND WHAT NOT TO EAT

The issue of what to eat when breaking your fast is made a lot easier thanks to following the keto diet regimen. This eliminates all sorts of harmful foods like sugary and processed food (think donuts, cakes, candy, etc.). The idea is to stay in ketosis, and thanks to the fasting period, your body will be in ketosis.

The amount of hunger you will feel depends on where you are in the process of adapting to the keto diet. Earlier in the process, when your body is still not burning fat as efficiently as possible, your cravings will combine with your hunger and make you ravenous.

Later on, though, you will feel what I like to think of as keto hunger. It will be a mild and less crazed version of the carb-fueled hunger. The main thing to remember at all times is to stay hydrated. Your body will be shedding water thanks to the lower carb intake, and it's easy to lose track of how much water you're drinking.

The next thing to keep in mind is your fiber intake. We've all grown up hating veggies in some form or another, but unless you want to earn a trip to the constipation zone, you will do well to eat your green leafy veggies! Make sure you're keeping up on your intake of fiber supplements that I'll talk about in the chapter on supplements.

Now that that's out of the way let's take a look at how you can break your fast in the best way possible and in a way that causes the least intrusion.

## Your First Meal

Here's the thing with the keto diet - you don't need to eat as much food in order to gain the same number of calories as with carbs. One gram of carbs releases four calories of energy, while one gram of fat released double that. Thus, a lot of people fall into the trap of feeling they're eating less and pile on more and more fat.

It's a good idea to visually train yourself by measuring out your meals and getting a feel for how much you ought to eat. It need not be accurate down to the last gram but in the ballpark. As you go on and gain more experience, you'll find that you'll start doing this automatically.

Now, the size of your first meal depends on when you've decided to work out. For those who have decided to work out fasted, this meal will be your largest, and you should consume 60% of your total calories in this meal, without a doubt. This will result in a large meal, but since you have not eaten anything since your workout, this point is non-negotiable.

For the rest, if you decide to work out immediately after the meal or after two meals, the first meal should have a healthy serving of protein and of course, fat. Make sure your protein content is high in this meal because your muscles have not been fed for a while, and your body is at a stage when it is beginning to think about possibly burning some muscle. Preempt this by feeding it with fat and bolstering your muscles with protein.

There is a lot of sense in having a lot of protein after your workout since this is what builds muscle. However, after your workout, there is zero chance of anything you eat being diverted to create fat, and almost everything goes towards nourishing and repairing your muscles (Berkhan, 2015).

Thus, as long as your protein content in the post workout meal is at a decent level, you'll be fine. It is far more critical, therefore, to feed your muscles coming out of the fasting period. Resist the urge to overeat, which will be strong in the initial days of your fast. As time goes on, your body will learn the new feeding regimen and will adjust its hunger hormone production accordingly.

### *Susan, How Do I Make This Easy?*

I get it. You're coming off a long period of not eating, and you're probably worried you'll go crazy and binge. Well, here's what you do. First, you whip up a large batch of keto bread and keto tortillas and keep them ready in the fridge.

Next, around an hour or so before you breaking your fast, get your protein ready. This meal could either be baked chicken breast or thighs. What I do is I keep a large batch of spicy homemade salsa ready to go. Once it's time, throw the baked chicken on the keto bread with some salsa, and you're good to go!

I have a sweet tooth, so I end the meal with a small piece of dark chocolate, and this keeps me going until my next meal, which is pretty similar calorie wise to the previous one. You can either switch it up to something else, maybe like canned tuna with mayo and then wait for your workout.

Speaking of canned tuna, it's a great option since it's high in protein, and by adding mayo and a touch of coconut or MCT oil, you get all the fat sustenance you need. Plus, it always works when you aren't in much of a mood to cook or you just plain forgot to do so.

By the way, if you're wondering what keto bread and keto tortillas are, worry not! The next section will give you the recipes for these fantastic staples. These will also go a long way towards giving your brain the impression you're eating carbs, so there's that benefit as well.

### *Keto Bread*

Ingredients:

- 6 large eggs
- 1/2 cup melted butter
- 1 tsp baking powder
- 2 tbsp coconut flour
- Salt

Recipe:

Place parchment paper on your loaf pan/medium baking pan. Preheat your oven to 400F.

Break the eggs into a bowl and start beating them

Gradually add the butter to the eggs. Once mixed well, slowly add the coconut flour, baking powder and salt to the mix.

Continue to beat well as the mixture thickens. If the mixture isn't thick enough to hang off your beater, then add some more flour.

Spread the mixture evenly in your loaf pan and place it in the oven.

Bake for forty minutes or until the bread is done. The best way to test for this is to insert a toothpick into the mixture. If it comes out clean, your bread is done.

Cool well and then cut into slices.

### *Keto Tortillas*

Ingredients:

- 4 large eggs

- 1 1/2 cup coconut milk

- 1/2 cup coconut flour

- Salt and pepper to taste

Recipe:

Break the eggs into a bowl and start beating them.

Begin making the batter by adding the coconut milk to the mix. Gradually add flour and salt and pepper. Keep beating until the consistency is to your liking.

Spread a little bit of the batter on a skillet and cook both sides until well done.

### *Other Alternatives*

Of course, this isn't the only way to do things. You could always cook up something fancier. There are several great keto recipes out there for keto fat bombs, coconut flakes, unsweetened cacao butter and so on. As long as you make sure your meal is in line with your overall caloric requirements, it's perfectly fine.

The beauty of the IF regimen you don't need to think twice about what you're eating, as long as you hit the broad guidelines. Even if you do make mistakes, which we all do, the fasting period acts as a leveler and ensures any excess calories are burned off.

This, of course, is not a license for you to eat whatever you want, as I've mentioned previously. You still need to work out your framework. IF helps when you stray slightly over the line, not completely obliterate it.

## *Supplements*

If you're training fasted early in the morning and maintaining a feeding window of 12:30-8 PM, then there is a bit of a gap until the first meal. It is essential that you consume the required amount of BCAA supplements as directed in the next chapter.

When breaking your fast, no matter which workout protocol you decide to follow, a protein shake is a good thing to consume since it gives you a quick boost of protein and the number of calories is also low. If you're having problems consuming less than 40% of your total calories and keeping the protein content high, add a scoop or two of protein powder.

If you're worried about what protein powder is, don't worry. I'll go over this in the next chapter.

So that's pretty much it. As you can see, there's no need to overthink the process of breaking your fast. All you need to do is align your workout schedule and your calorie consumption accordingly. Typing that previous sentence was more complicated than actually doing what it says.

Make sure you're well stocked up on your staples, and whipping up a quick and delicious meal will be a cinch!

# CHAPTER 4:

## HOW TO EXERCISE WHEN FASTING ON KETO (*WITHOUT KILLING YOURSELF!*)

Exercise is hard, and for a good reason. If you don't put your body under some stress, you can never hope to make any progress. Exercise is also intimidating. No, I'm not talking about the gym bros and the swimsuit models that invariably seem to work out only when you choose to.

I mean that there's so much information out there that the exercise industry is just as screwed up as the diet industry is. I mean, why is it this hard to get fit? In this chapter, I'll clear all this up for you and give you a clear plan to move forward with.

Even if you don't find it to your liking, don't worry. I'll give you a framework within which you can design your workout routine and get fit in the healthiest way possible!

# EXERCISE BASICS

Before I get into the different types of workouts and timing considerations, it's necessary to step back and understand some basics. To avoid the need to repeat myself and explain terms, I'll be using and also because this stuff should be general knowledge but is presented in such a muddled manner in the mainstream media that it confuses everyone.

Generally speaking, there are two primary ways of exercising: Strength training and Cardio. Cardio stands for cardiovascular training, and cardiovascular refers to the system of the same name within you, which encompasses your lungs, heart, and a few other organs. Strength training builds your anaerobic performance, whereas cardio builds your aerobic performance.

Anaerobic refers to your ability to complete tasks without or with very little oxygen. Think of lifting something heavy off the floor. We generally hold our breath and tighten ourselves as much as possible to generate strength. Aerobic exercise refers to your performance when oxygen is available, but you need to perform the activity over longer periods.

Running, swimming, hiking, and cycling are prime examples of aerobic activity. Your performance in these tasks doesn't depend as much on your strength as it does on your heart's ability to keep pumping oxygen-rich blood over long periods of time.

Now that we've got the basic definitions out of the way let's dig deeper.

## Anaerobic Exercise

Anaerobic exercise is what you see, most of the time, being performed in the gym. Which involves the lifting of weights a set number of times for a certain number of repetitions. Now, it is possible to train your cardio system using weights, but it is an inefficient use of your time. It's a bit like using a bicycle to try to win a two-wheeler race. Yes, you can technically do it, but you're probably better off trying to win on a motorbike.

When training with weights, your primary aim should be to increase your strength. Strength training helps directly build more muscle in your body, and the more muscle you have, the stronger you are. Apart from being able to lift heavier stuff, your increased muscle mass has another side effect. Your body will have less of a need to store fat.

Fat storage amounts are determined by the body using this logic. If you're weak, in case a crisis like a famine or a drought hits, you're more vulnerable to it. In other words, your chances of dying are high, and therefore, you need higher levels of emergency fuel, which is fat. If you're stronger, your body reasons that you can make it out of the crisis better, and in this case, you don't need as much fat.

That is why people who are lean can get away with eating anything they want for short periods of time. Their bodies are accustomed to converting and feeding their muscles, so by this point, it pretty much shovels everything into muscle, no matter how rubbish it might be. A great example of this was Michael Phelps back when he was winning gold medals seemingly every day.

As a part of his diet, he was consuming close to 10,000 calories per day in the form of high cholesterol, fatty, and processed food. He could get away with it because his training regimen as an Olympic swimmer demanded so much energy that his body took whatever it could get. Olympic sprinters, too, tend to consume a lot of junk food occasionally.

My point is, once you're lean, you can break more rules. However, you cannot break them for a long time and expect to get away with it. The stronger you are, that is, the more muscle you have, the better your chances of wolfing down that entire cheesecake and still having your abs show.

Strength training can be divided into three categories:

- Low rep/high weight

- Medium rep/medium weight

- High rep/low weight

Rep here stands for repetitions, that is the number of times you lift weight in a particular exercise. A set is a set of reps. So if you perform an exercise for three sets of five reps, you'll be lifting weight five times, three times each.

For strength building purposes, low rep/high weight is generally the best. That is because the weight is at its heaviest here, and you'll reach your strength limits sooner. Pushing your strength limits is a good thing because this is how you can increase your overall strength. A low rep count would be anything up to five or six reps.

Medium rep/medium weight is best for building strength and attaining a great shape. Over this rep range, a phenomenon called hypertrophy occurs, which gives your muscles excellent shape and doesn't happen with lower reps. With medium reps, you can also better isolate and work on individual muscles. A medium rep range would be anywhere from six to fifteen reps.

High reps can be used for cardio purposes. Performing full body movements like the squat or bench press for these many reps will get your heart pumping quick. However, you're better off spending your time doing cardio than high reps for this purpose. You will sometimes see bodybuilders perform high rep counts with extremely low weight, to give their muscles better aesthetics for competition. As such, you need not concern yourself with this.

So, which one should you follow? Well, if you've never worked out in a gym before, you're best off starting with low reps. I'll give you a list of exercises you can perform here shortly, so don't worry about designing a training program. Too many beginners jump into the medium rep range and don't see the results they want.

Here's the thing. To build aesthetics, you need to have a baseline of strength, which is really muscle. If you don't have this, all you're doing is toning your fat. If you skip a week at the gym, all that fat is simply going to lose its tightness and jiggle again. What you need to be doing is replacing that fat with muscle, which is what low rep ranges will do.

### *Exercise Program*

There are several fantastic beginner strength training programs out there. The most popular one is the Starting Strength 3X5 method, which represents the sets and reps you need to perform. Another popular program is the Stronglifts 5X5 program, which is pretty much the same as Starting Strength save for the number of sets you need to perform.

Both these programs are designed the same way. They center around the back squat as the main exercise and rotate the bench press, overhead press, deadlift, and barbell row around it. You will be working out thrice a week for an hour at the most. Anything more than this is overkill, given the physical demands of these exercises.

You can find details for the programs at startingstrength.com and stronglifts.com. Both websites are excellent resources, and they give you a weekly workout plan. It's pretty simple really - you squat thrice a week and perform two out of the remaining exercises.

It is crucial that you master the correct techniques for these exercises before increasing the weight. Given that all of these movements are compound ones, in other words, you'll be using muscles from all over your body; bad form will lead to injury. So set your ego aside and learn proper form.

Here's another thing that will happen, and I might as well let you know now. You will be the only girl in your gym doing these exercises. You see, mainstream fitness advice has convinced us, women, that we need to stick to small weights and exercise bikes. Well, this is complete nonsense! Go ahead and wander over to the heavyweight area where all these exercises are usually done and stick to your routine. You'll find the more serious lifters over there will come by and give you tips and compliments - trust me.

Both the exercise programs mentioned above have certain strength standards by which you can mark your progress. Once you reach an intermediate level of strength, you can then either continue with the programs or switch to a split routine. A split refers to training different parts of your body on different days.

Generally, split routines are nowhere near as taxing as compound movements, since you're recruiting fewer muscles, but it will help target and increase strength in certain areas. With a proper split routine, you can cut down on the compound movements' frequency and find your performance on them gets better.

Bodybuilding.com is an excellent resource for split routines and to be honest, by the time you reach this level, you'll know what to look for. Aim to train for four days a week at the least, and hit all areas of your body. Incorporate one compound movement per workout. So squat one day, bench the next, followed by the overhead press on the third and deadlift on the fourth day.

One important point to note here is that before starting your strength training programs, buy yourself a good pair of flat soled shoes. Ditch the gel-filled Nikes and Asics, which are only good for running. For lifting weights, you need your feet firmly planted on the floor.

You might be wondering where cardio fits into all of this or if you should even be doing it. Well, let's look at this next.

## *Aerobic Exercise*

It's always a good idea to perform some form of aerobic exercise after your workout. If you're used to running or swimming, though, I have some bad news for you. At this point, it is best for you to focus on building your strength. The thing with all forms of cardio is that they will build your strength up to a certain point, but not beyond that.

To perform better in your aerobic activities, you need better anaerobic performance. Think of it this way: if your body can perform anaerobically well, then it needs to divert lesser amounts of oxygen than usual to sustain it once the anaerobic activity is done. In other words, you'll be huffing and puffing less.

Keep your aerobic exercise to a maximum of fifteen minutes after your workout. Do not perform cardio before your workout, since this will deplete your strength and you will not build as much muscle as you can. It will seem odd to you at first if you're used to only performing cardio, but stick with it, and you'll soon see how much better your cardio performance gets.

So what sort of cardio should you do? Well, anything that you like, to be honest. Running, Zumba, dance classes, whatever floats your boat. The only requirement of cardio is that you need to break a sweat and move. As long as you achieve this, you'll be fine. As you begin to lift heavier weights in your strength training routine, you'll find yourself less inclined to perform cardio.

If you feel completely exhausted, don't push yourself. It's perfectly fine if you miss a day's worth of cardio and only do it twice a week. It's far more important for you to train for strength.

You will read or might have read by now that cardio is great for fat loss. Well, actually, yes it is. However, if you perform only cardio, you will hit a fat loss plateau and then stop losing more weight. The reason for this is that, as I mentioned before, cardio builds your strength up to a certain limit.

As long as your strength is being built up, you will lose fat. Once you hit this strength limit, there's no reason for your body to shed fat anymore, unless you ramp up your cardio to insane levels and force your body to burn it off.

The long and short of all this is: focus on building strength and muscle and limit your cardio to fifteen minutes post-workout.

## *HIIT*

High-intensity interval training, or HIIT, is an alternative to cardio which has gained enormous popularity. HIIT, despite being a form of cardio, it's an anaerobic form of exercise where you push yourself to the absolute limit for a short interval and then rest for a slightly longer interval. Then, you push again, and so on for around fifteen to twenty minutes.

That's fifteen to twenty minutes without strength training, mind you. Usual steady state cardio, such as cycling or swimming, needs to be performed for close to forty-five minutes (without strength training) to have a positive effect on your fitness. With HIIT, you can cut this down in half and still reap the benefits.

So which activities can you do with HIIT? Pretty much anything! The only requirement is that you push yourself to the absolute limit. Traditional HIIT intervals are set up as one minute of work and two minutes of rest, following this pattern for fifteen or twenty minutes.

As your performance increases, you keep reducing the size of your rest intervals until you're working for a minute and resting for half a minute. A popular HIIT training method is to sprint and then walk or jog, with the sprint making up the work interval. Alternatively, you could skip rope or work the stationary bike at your gym. Swimming is not recommended for HIIT since there is the chance you could drown due to exhaustion. Neither is cycling on the road due to the dangers of traffic.

So how should you integrate HIIT into your routine, should you so choose? Well, first off, if you're doing HIIT, you don't need to perform cardio. I'm saying this because you're already doing a lot of work via strength training and you'll exhaust yourself doing things this way.

Next, don't perform HIIT after your workout. Instead, designate a separate day to do this and spend up to twenty minutes on your HIIT routine. Once you're past the beginner stage, experiment with what feels better and implement it accordingly.

So, now that you have learned the basics let's see how you can implement an exercise routine within the IF framework.

## EXERCISE OPTIONS

As mentioned previously, you have three choices when it comes to working out. You can either work out fasted, after one meal, or at least two meals. I previously discouraged you from adopting the fasted training routine since it is incredibly taxing. However, given that it is the one which will give you the most rapid results, it's worth taking a look at.

## *Fasted Training*

When I say fasted training, I'm going to assume you wake up early in the morning, and before getting ready for work or your household duties, you get a workout in. If, like most people, you're going to be breaking your fast around 12:30 PM, this is a problem since you will not be eating before or after your workout.

The problem with working out fasted is that you will burn muscle once your energy stores are depleted. What's more, if you don't replenish your muscles post workout, you're going to lose even more muscle mass. So all that lifting during your workout isn't worth squat.

You solve this problem via supplements, specifically BCAA supplements. BCAA stands for branch chain amino acids, and they contain the stuff that muscles and protein are literally made of. You need to take 10g BCAA 15 minutes before working out, 10g an hour after, and another 10g every two hours until you break your fast (Berkhan, 2015). That is pretty much the protocol Martin Berkhan recommends on his leangains website.

At first, you will feel odd not eating something after working out, but this is just your body reacting to your pattern up until now. Eventually, you'll find that your body will adjust to the new regimen. Just remember that the meal you break your fast with should be the largest of the day, with over 60% of your calorie intake occurring here.

Try to avoid HIIT training in a fasted state. HIIT demands an extreme amount of glycogen from your body, and performing this fasted might leave you with hypoglycemic conditions. Again, if you perform HIIT once or twice, it shouldn't be an issue. Just don't make a habit of it.

### *Training After One or Multiple Meals*

The protocols for training after one or multiple meals are pretty much the same. You need to follow the guidelines for eating the right amount of calories per meal, with the majority of the 60% coming during your post-workout meal. Other than this, it is just a question of timing and aligning your meals with the rest of your workday.

The only time this protocol is shifted is during your rest days. That is when you will not be working out. During such days, the meal with which you break your fast should be your largest.

### *Which One Should I Follow?*

I prefer working out towards the end of the workday and having my last meal end my feeding period. This way, I have a couple of hours or so until bedtime and am good and ready to go to sleep. There's no better sleep than the one you experience after a tough workout.

Of course, life is different for every one of us, so you should think about this long and hard. Adjusting the feeding window might be an option if you wish to avoid fasted workouts. However, if you begin eating at 7 AM, you'll have to wrap things up by 3 PM, which is a bit awkward in terms of timing.

It is a lot easier to skip breakfast than it is to skip dinner since it is psychologically difficult to go to bed on an empty stomach. I recommend the 12-8 window. Don't be afraid of supplements or think they're steroids of some kind. All supplements recommended in this book are perfectly safe and legal to consume. None of them will enhance you in any way that regular food won't.

Thus, if early morning fasted training is the only way for you to move forward, then so be it. You will need to prep additionally for the BCAA and make sure you're well stocked. I'll address the different types of protein you can consume in the supplements chapter, but for fasted workouts stick to BCAA.

There may be some of you who will be wondering whether it is OK to exercise after the feeding window closes, or late at night? Well, no. It isn't. It is imperative to feed your body with protein both before and after your workout.

If you work out at night, effectively beginning your fasting phase with a workout, you'll guarantee that muscle will burn along with fat. After a workout, muscles deteriorate thanks to the strain they've been placed under. Supplying them with protein is how they repair themselves and get stronger.

So, as you can see, depriving your body of nutrition is not a good idea post workout. With the fasted workout, you keep the deterioration at bay since you consume BCAA, which is a fast-acting protein. Then, with your first meal being the largest, you can provide whole food to your muscles. That is not the case for a late night workout.

The final factor you should consider when deciding to work out is the level of fatigue you will encounter. Initially, with both the strength training programs I've recommended, you will not feel a lot of strain. However, as time goes on, roughly around the end of the first month, those weights are going to start to feel heavy.

If you haven't checked out the programs as yet, basically, you need to keep increasing the weight you lift every workout. This way, even if you stall a few times, within three months, you'll be near an intermediate level of strength, not to mention you will look entirely different.

The negative side of this is the mental toll lifting such constantly increasing weight takes. While you'll feel great, the workouts themselves and your post workout state will be one of exhaustion. Thus, it's best to leave it for the last thing in the day, right before your final meal. This way, you ensure you get great sleep as well as go to bed on a full stomach.

## THE KETO EFFECT

Since you'll be following the keto diet while implementing the IF protocol, there are additional things you need to be aware of. First off, once you reduce your carb intake, your glycogen stores are going to be depleted. Once your body is fully adjusted to the new diet, it won't need too much glycogen to keep around as spare since it's perfectly capable of using fat now.

I mentioned in the earlier chapter that during the first week, it's best not to work out since your body will be adjusting to the new diet. By workout, I don't mean to say don't perform any physical activity whatsoever. Feel free to do some light cardio or even regular cardio.

Adopting the keto diet is going to impact your anaerobic performance, and you will find making gains in the gym difficult beyond a certain point. Furthermore, since you're on a caloric deficit, this is the worst of both worlds if your aim is to gain muscle fast. Now, there's a difference between having a goal of fat loss versus gaining muscle even though one implies the other.

If you wish to gain muscle, you need to maintain a caloric excess, which is to eat more than you need. Carbs help the muscle building process thank to the glycogen they provide. Glycogen is the body's priority as fuel due to the fact that it can burn immediately and provide instant energy.

Fat takes a bit longer to burn and thus, in situations where you need instant performance, as is the case in anaerobic activity, you will feel a drop in performance. I don't mean to say you won't be able to lift anything. It's just that you will make slower progress and will stall at certain levels faster.

Stalling refers to when your strength plateaus and you cannot go past a certain level. The way to get around this is to reduce the weight slightly and then attack the level again. Both starting strength and strong lifts go into detail with regards to handling stalls, so don't worry about this too much.

Just remember that your performance with cardio is going to be better than with strength training. That doesn't mean you should ignore strength training since your cardio is 'better.' In fact, it means the exact opposite, since by expending more energy on strength training, you'll burn more fat off your body.

Is there a way to get the best of both worlds? To have glycogen available but still follow the keto diet? Well, this is what the TKD and CKD are. However, following these diet protocols requires a lot of prep and calculation, not to mention maintenance. For anyone with a full-time job, this is akin to taking another job if you're not terribly passionate about dieting and fitness.

If this is your cup of tea, though, try experimenting with it. What you can do is consume up to fifteen grams of high GI carbs like bananas or white potatoes pre-workout, while keeping your overall carb count under thirty grams or forty. That's fifteen grams of carbs by the way, not fifteen grams of potatoes. Doing this will give you a boost headed into your workout, and you will be able to use this energy to fuel your lifts.

Just make sure your workouts are of high intensity, and then track how long it takes you to get back into ketosis via the methods I'll show you in the chapter on tracking.

So, this concludes the section on exercise. For the first time, you have some homework to do! Go ahead and check out Starting Strength or Stronglifts and understand how the routines work. They're pretty straight forward, I promise.

Once you've drawn up the routines, figure out when you can work out during your work day and how you'll need to schedule your meals, as detailed in this chapter and the prep chapter.

There will be some confusion about all of this. The next chapter will address this via a bunch of do's and don'ts you need to be aware of.

# CHAPTER 5:

## THE DO'S AND DON'TS
## YOU MUST BE AWARE OF

If this is your first-time dieting or if you're relatively inexperienced, this whole IF plus keto thing is going to take some adjusting. Mainly because we're looking to combine two methods into a single, efficient one. Even if you have dieted before, you will recall the difficulties you had when first implementing it and the steps you had to take to overcome those difficulties.

Well, this chapter is going to serve as a primer for what to do and what not to do with everything that is going on here. It will help to check back in with this chapter to see if you're following everything correctly.

For simplicity's sake, I've divided the do's and don'ts into three sections, namely, intermittent fasting, ketogenic diet, and exercise guidelines. This way, any questions you have can be answered quickly and easily. So, without further ado, let's look at the things you need to do and those you should watch out for regarding intermittent fasting!

## IF DO'S AND DON'TS

Let's begin with the things you should do first.

### *Health*

Are you pregnant? Under eighteen? Are you taking prescription medicine? All or any of the above? Well, if that is the case, you should not be fasting. Always make sure to check with your doctor before making any changes to your diet. While intermittent fasting is the fastest way to get healthy and lose fat, it isn't the only way.

A good approach for you to take is to clean your diet of chemically processed food and things that are high in sugar. More than anything else, these two factors will go a long way in making sure you get healthy. Chemically processed items include things like store-bought frozen pizza, highly processed oils, and so on.

Drink water as much as possible and cut down on alcohol, and you'll be doing yourself a huge favor. Eating clean may not bring the immediate benefits that IF does, but over time, the results will show. All you need to do is stick with it.

## *Lifestyle*

The biggest challenge you will face when adopting a new diet or fitness regimen is to fit it into your lifestyle, and it's no different with IF. Common concerns include social ones as well as mental blocks against skipping meals, etc. From a social standpoint, skipping breakfast is the easiest way to do this, but if you like hanging out late with friends and such, you will find it difficult to say no to those late night snacks.

So, make sure you have a plan of action before these events. Take into account that when you're staying up late, the hunger will seem more significant because you're awake when usually the majority of your hunger occurs when asleep.

The biggest hurdle regarding breakfast as being the most important meal of the day is technically correct if your last meal happens to be at 6 PM. If you wake up at 6 AM, that's a twelve-hour gap, and, logically, you need to eat something.

Well, with IF, your final meal is going to be a lot later than 6 PM, and there's also the fact that your body can run longer than you think without food. So stop treating yourself as a weakling and just do it!

## What's Your Why?

Why are you doing this? What benefits do you expect to accrue by doing so? How will your life be better, and which goals will you reach by following through on this?

*(Knowing all of this before implementing IF is crucial for your success.)*

As you've seen by now, IF requires work, and that's without the keto and exercising part. Over and above, you'll be in a caloric deficit. So why are you doing this? Keep it written somewhere handy so that you can remind yourself at all times.

## Moderation in Exercise

You need to train hard but know the difference between training hard and going for broke. Your body is in a stressed state, and while this is good for it, too much of it will lead to the production of cortisol. Cortisol is a hormone that is produced as part of the stress response and ultimately will lead to you gaining fat.

A rule of thumb is to leave a rep or two in the tank when working out, instead of going until failure. Going to failure on the odd set is perfectly fine, but don't do it every single time. The same goes for HIIT. Don't overdo it beyond the single day per week, and don't do it while fasted.

## Supplements

Vitamins, minerals, and other supplements play an essential role in helping you with IF. During the fasted state, you will experience micronutrient loss, which you'll need to wait until the feeding period to replenish. Stock up on the necessary vitamins and make sure you're getting a good dose of them.

I'll talk about this in detail in the chapter on supplements.

## Fun

Look, it doesn't have to be dreary all the time. Schedule something relaxing or fun to do during your fasted state during the weekend or if you happen to be free. Massages are my go-to secret weapon against fasted state ennui. Book yourself a session at the spa and pamper yourself. Not only will you be treating yourself, but you'll also be getting healthier while doing so!

During your downtime, steer clear of any food or hunger triggers. Don't go shopping for food when you're in the fasted state, and certainly don't watch cooking or food shows in this state. Just be smart and help yourself towards your goal!

## *Recruit Help*

Why not talk your friend into doing this, too? If your friend isn't too keen, then sign up for forums online and join Facebook groups. There are a many of resources out there for support and help, so don't be shy to introduce yourself and get help.

Everyone struggles with new diets, so don't expect yourself to be an exception. Go ahead and recruit someone to help support you and do the same for them.

Now, here's a list of the things you should NOT do before implementing IF

## *Ignore Your Doctor*

If you experience something out of the ordinary, according to you or anyone else, let your doctor know. If you have any doubts about all of this, then ask your doctor. If you have any questions about how some of your health conditions might be affected, ask your doctor.

You get the idea. Do not neglect to inform your doctor about what you're doing. Keep them updated and follow their advice always.

## *Last Supper Syndrome*

You're not going to jail or the guillotine. You're just eating differently. You don't need to think of this as some sort of purgatory, all right? So, put down that cheesecake and eat as you regularly would the day before you begin your new diet.

A lot of people sabotage themselves before they even begin. Think about it: if you think of your diet as being a jail of some sort, why would you want to be in it? Why would you want to follow its rules? When was the last time you intentionally sabotaged yourself, when fully conscious?

Stop making things harder for yourself and be reasonable about all of this. It is not a big deal. You've prepared and are fully ready for it.

## *I'm Tough!!*

A lot of us women feel the need to prove ourselves as being physically strong and competent. After all, society tells us we're weak and that the heavy lifting is what men do. Well, you need not try to be a hero and prove all the doubters wrong.

Some women take it too far by pushing too hard and too fast in the gym. Examples of this would be trying to compete with the big dude squatting next to you - except he's been doing it for years now with perfect form, and you've just begun. All you'll get out of this is a sprained knee.

This way of thinking is an insidious form of self-sabotage since it cloaks within self-improvement garb. Be on the lookout for this and follow the guidelines I've given you in this book.

### Ignore Hydration

Water is the seed of life. Or something like that. You will lose water in copious amounts both during your fasted period as well as thanks to the keto regimen, so make sure to hydrate. Also, just as an aside, you don't need one of those ridiculous apps to track how much water you've been drinking all day.

You know when you're thirsty and drink when you feel so. Is your pee yellow? Drink water. Mind you, if you're going to be taking multivitamins, your pee will be yellow-tinged. A better indication is monitoring how often you need to pee. If you need to go every hour, you're probably drinking too much.

Is your head hurting? Are you feeling dizzy? Then drink some water ASAP.

### Add Stress

Life can be tough. If it gets too tough, don't force yourself to go work out, which is likely to stress you out further and might push you off your diet. If you feel tired and want to sleep, go ahead and do so. Remember, the diet is more important than the workout.

If you feel tired during the workout and don't feel like you can continue, stop exercising. There's no gain in harming yourself - work within your limits. Schedule some massages and indulge in some weekend yoga to relieve your stress.

## KETO DO'S AND DON'TS

The keto diet is a bit more challenging mentally as compared to the IF protocol since we're so used to eating carbs all the time. Added to this is the initial keto fog that everyone goes through, and you have a perfect recipe for breaking your rules. The good news is that a lot of the do's and don'ts carry over from the previous section. Thus, I'll cover the stuff that is keto specific.

Let's begin with the things you should be doing.

### *Whole Food*

It'll be tempting to take shortcuts and eat chemically processed food that is high in fat. Avoid this temptation and clean up your diet. What I mean by this is you need to stick to real food like cheese, butter, etc. and avoid the processed stuff like marmalade and margarine.

Similarly, when it comes to meat, stick to whole lean cuts instead of minced meat, which tends to be a mixture of unwanted stuff like bone and cartilage. It's fine to buy frozen meat for cost considerations. Just stay away from pre-packaged, cooked meals that don't need refrigeration and can last for months on end.

## Hydrate!

Yes, I know I've covered this, but it bears repeating. Always hydrate! Powerade doesn't count, even after the gym! Well, it will hydrate you, but you might as well drink sugar mixed with water for the good it'll do you.

Stick to good ol' water, and you'll be just fine. Follow the instructions from the previous section (Ignoring Hydration) for tips on monitoring your hydration levels. Another excellent option is to consume chicken or beef stock. Bone broth is another option which has gained popularity, but since you'll be cooking chicken and beef, the former might be better options.

## Eat That Fat!

All our lives, we've been conditioned to remove fat from our diets and avoid things which are high in fat. The keto diet turns this belief on its head, and it's not going to be easy to switch overnight. You need to consciously be aware of what food you're preparing and eating.

If you don't like the marble on your meat, that's fine. However, don't subconsciously cut down on butter or cream.

Stick to your portions, as per the calorie counts you did previously, and eat that quantity, this also applies equally to cooking oils. There's a lot of stuff available that are advertised as low fat and low cholesterol and so on. All the while, the healthy stuff, like olive oil and coconut oil, sits behind one of these fancy oils.

A word of caution: there is a type of oil called olive pomace oil, which you need to stay away from, as much as possible, stick to extra virgin or virgin olive oil. Extra virgin oil is what is extracted from the first cold press of the olives. Virgin is what comes on the second press.

Pomace oil is chemically extracted from the husks of the olives and is not much different from any processed oil. However, thanks to advertising standards, it is sold as olive oil and tends to be a lot cheaper than the good stuff. Stay away from this. If you want a cheaper oil, try coconut oil.

Given the high-fat quantities of these oils, you'll need less of them to cook with, so the cost will even out in the long run.

In addition to pomace oil, stay away from canola, corn, vegetable, peanut, and soy oil. A good rule of thumb is to stick to cold pressed oils. Cold pressed refers to the source of the oil being pressed to extract the oil within it. A hot press usually involves some form of chemical extraction.

## *Go Easy on Sweeteners*

One of the drawbacks of the keto diet is the complete lack of anything sweet. Given the ban on sugar, if you have a sweet tooth, this can be a problem. Here's the good news: Once you remove sugar from your diet, you'll be amazed at how satisfied you will be with the tiniest hint of something sweet.

Even things like dark chocolate mixed with peanut butter will not taste as bitter to you. On the keto diet, you can use sweeteners but stick to the natural ones like Stevia and Erythritol. Mind you, consuming these in excess is bad as well, so you need to exercise your willpower and minimize them.

## *Avoid Fast Food*

I mean, this is just good health advice, not keto specific. If you're going to eat clean, giving fast food, the heave-ho is a no brainer. Sometimes, you'll be pressed for time and will have to resort to it. If you do choose to go this way occasionally or for your cheat meal, then minimize the damage as much as possible.

Opt for burgers without the bun and so on. However, even the meat is of poor quality; usually, just cheap mince bound together, so it's not like there's any great nutritional value there.

### *Know What You're Eating*

Eating something and then trying to figure out how many calories and macros you've eaten is doing things backward. Always measure your food out before you eat it and know whether or not your calorie requirements are being met.

In restaurants, this will be a problem, and no one wants to be the Karen who bores the manager with questions about the exact nutritional value of the food being cooked. Here's a simple method to follow: have as much protein as you can. Eating additional protein is not a problem. You're already avoiding the carbs, so that shouldn't be an issue.

Minimize the fat you're eating. Instead of spooning the entire cup of butter, have just half. Over time, as you get used to your portion sizes, you'll be able to estimate or feel how much is the appropriate amount. In the beginning, though, stick to protein as much as possible.

### *Add Seeds and Nuts*

Want a quick and easy snack? Add a mixture of nuts and seeds to your diet and carry them around with you. Be careful, though. It's easy to eat too much fat with these since they're so small and you can lose track of how much you've had.

Next time you watch a movie, pack some nuts instead of starving yourself as people around you gorge themselves on popcorn.

To round things off, here's a simple don't for you:

### *"Sugar-Free"*

I'm not going to bore you on the veracity of these labels, but generally speaking, stay away from these types of products. Just because something is labeled sugar free doesn't mean it is healthy for you. Organic is another labeling con job that occurs frequently.

The key to all of this is to stick to natural, whole food as much as possible. If you're buying eggs, buy the ones which are labeled free-range or organic (despite my previous misgivings). Stay away from the 'omega 3' eggs, similarly with vegetables and other produce.

Keto dishes are straightforward to put together since, for the most part. It's just protein with salad and a little sauce drizzled over it or cheese/butter on the side. All of that stuff is natural food and doesn't come with processed junk in it or a bunch of labels on it.

# EXERCISE DO'S AND DON'TS

The lists for keto and IF overlap quite a bit so if you follow one, the other pretty much takes care of itself. But that's not the case when it comes to exercising, though. I understand that a lot of you will not have stepped foot inside a gym in your lives previously, and this fine. There's a first time for everything.

So, without further ado, here's what you should be doing in the gym.

## *Lack of Prep*

Do you know what your workout plan is? Are you maintaining a journal with the list of exercises you need to do on that day and tracking them? Or are you deciding on the spot that you'll lift this and do that?

Remember, you need to plan things ahead of time, this will include your training routine and what it is you're going to be doing in the gym. A lot of people treat the gym as a punishment of sorts and end up walking on the treadmill while watching TV.

Don't be one of these mopes! The reason they get bored is that they haven't planned anything out or thought things through. It'll be tough at first, but make sure you plan everything about your workout, from warm-ups to finishing exercises. Speaking of warm-ups...

## *Always Warm Up*

Not warming up is the easiest way to end up with a sprain or a pulled muscle of some sort. The best warm-ups are those that get your body temperature up but don't leave you sweating profusely and gasping for air. Walking for a few minutes at a brisk pace followed by some light yoga is a perfect warm up.

Skipping rope is also a great way to get yourself going. Another aspect of warming up is to ramp up your lifts. Warming up will not be a problem at first since you'll be lifting less weight, but as you progress, you will need to build up to your work set level. A good rule of thumb is to do five sets of warm-ups, beginning with the lowest weight and then working your way up to the weight you lifted successfully two or three workouts ago.

The aim of the ramped warm up is to let your body know that some heavyweight is coming and that it needs to get ready, this is especially true of squats. Once you've warmed up at the start of your workout, you don't need to ramp into your remaining lifts. Lift the planned weight.

## *Compound Your Lifts*

Focus on building muscle first and then worry about sculpting your body. The best way to build muscle is to employ compound lifts like the squat, deadlift, etc. These lifts recruit almost every muscle in your body and develop what I like to think of as muscle connectivity.

In other words, your muscles learn to work with one another efficiently. So the next time you pick something up off the floor, it won't be just your back taking the load - your posterior chain and core will come to the rescue as well.

## *Learn Proper Form*

I can't overstate this enough. Without proper form, your lifts are useless. What's more, with compound lifts, you risk major injury if you don't follow proper form. Always start with the least amount of weight and don't get caught up with endlessly increasing weight.

Remember, the goal is increased weight as long as you can maintain proper form. Learn the exercises, and if you're having problems, consider hiring a trainer to help you out with these movements. Take your time with the lower weights, and once you master them, move on to higher weight while keeping an eye out for your form.

Breaking form for a rep or two on your final set is fine, since you're pushing for higher gains and will probably be tired. You need to achieve that balance between pushing hard and relaxing your form on those tough reps and being absolutly strict to form.

## *Rest*

Discipline is something you will need if you are to be successful. What a lot of people don't realize, however, is that in addition to doing certain things are certain times, such as pushing yourself to exercise, you also need to stay put and do nothing, like rest when you should.

In the beginning, the weight you lift is not going to be too heavy, and you'll feel as if your rest periods are unnecessary. The strength training programs I mentioned call for a rest day in between the three workout days. So, at first, you'll feel as if the rest days are not of much use and will be tempted to advance your workout.

Do not do this. True, you might not need the rest, but the reason you need to follow the routine is to build discipline. If you violate it right from the start, when the weights do get heavy, you'll set yourself up for not going to the gym at all and missing your goals. Hence, do it right from the start.

Speaking of being tired, if you feel exhausted and like you're unable to lift anything, go to the gym anyway and try to lift something. If you feel tired after this, then it's fine to skip that workout. If need be, take a week off and then get back to it. Taking breaks is a good thing, and don't let the specter of discipline throw you off course.

During your workout, make sure you take adequate rest between your sets and don't rush yourself. You need to maintain proper form, and enough rest between sets is the best way to do this.

## Intensity

Make sure you maintain a good intensity with your workouts. This means take rest, but not too much rest between sets, which will result in your heart rate decreasing. However, a good intensity doesn't mean you need to be panting all the time either.

So, find your sweet spot and stay there.

Here are the things you should NOT do when it comes to training

## Worry About Anyone Else

No one is looking at you or passing any judgment, so stop worrying about this. Yes, you will make mistakes, but so have all the other man mountains around you. Calm down and focus on what you need to do. Far too many women let their self-consciousness interfere with the task at hand and end up sabotaging themselves.

Don't be one of them.

## Comparisons

It will be tempting when you're lifting an empty bar to look over and see the gym bros next to you pumping out squats with all the plates in the gym on his bar and wistfully wonder if you'll ever get there.

Look, comparing yourself to someone else gets you nowhere. I know this is extremely hard advice to follow in a gym, but seriously, don't do it. Practice some self-love and remind yourself of your goals regularly and how hard you're working to achieve them.

Always be kind and compassionate to yourself, and the results are sure to follow.

## Doing Too Much

It will be tempting to do everything: strength training, cardio, and HIIT, all at once in an attempt to achieve maximum fat loss. Remember always to rest when you need to and keep things simple. Remember what I said about discipline above.

## I Don't Want That Bulk!

Bulking has to be the most nonsensical fear that women have. I'll say it again: you will not end up looking like a dude just from lifting weights! If anything, you will look more feminine because of the way your features will be highlighted.

Unless you choose to juice up on steroids or any such unnatural thing, you will look just fine. And no, you won't end up looking like those female bodybuilders either. So relax and put your plan in action.

## A FINAL NOTE

Sudden weight loss will affect your menstrual cycle, and there are some anecdotal stories of women being affected by this (Berkhan, 2015). If you maintain a healthy deficit of 500 calories per day, then you should not have any such issues. If you do have such issues, then you're probably losing too much weight too fast.

The reason for this is that your deficit is too high. Now, your deficit is made of two components: one is the amount of food you're eating, and the second is the energy you're burning. If your workouts are too strenuous, then dial it back a bit and see if it changes anything.

If your workouts aren't particularly intense and you're still losing weight, then you're just not eating enough. Increase your calorie count by 500 calories and see how that changes things. Ultimately, if nothing works, see your doctor and follow what they recommend.

# CHAPTER 6:

## TIPS AND TRICKS FOR MOMS

Every woman who's had kids has been there. That post-pregnancy weight refuses to budge, and you barely have any time now that you need to take care of your little one. It's a tough period for any woman and while your desire to lose weight is high, should you go ahead and implement an IF plus keto regimen?

Well, first off, it needs to be said that if you're pregnant, you should not be fasting for any reason whatsoever (Berkhan, 2015). Fasting will put both you and your baby in harm's way. As for the keto diet, it depends. Let's start by looking at this first.

## KETO WHEN PREGNANT

The truth of the matter is that there isn't any conclusive research on the subject due to almost no study enrolling pregnant women out of ethical concerns. Furthermore, one of the tests your doctor will conduct is to check for ketoacidosis, which is the presence of excessive ketones in your urine and blood (Kubala, 2018).

Ketoacidosis is an extremely bad sign and will result in pregnancy complications. If you're on the keto diet, then you will be producing ketones. So how much is a good level? Well, again, it depends on your doctor. The more conservative ones will advise you to not take any chances for fear of missing harmful symptoms over regular ketones (Kubala, 2018).

Some doctors are comfortable with this, however. Indeed, some doctors even advise beginning the keto diet two to three months before you try to get pregnant since you'll be fat-adapted by the time your baby is conceived (Mullens & Dr. Andreas Eenfeldt, 2019). Doctors report reduced rates of miscarriages, preeclampsia, and morning sickness when adopting the keto diet.

What is not recommended is changing your diet once you become pregnant. Ultimately, the best thing you can do is to speak to your doctor and let them know all about your diet and lifestyle. Follow what they say, and you'll be fine. You can always lose that weight once your baby is delivered.

Different bodies run on different types of nutrition, with some resistant to carbs and some preferring fat. So, check with your doctor and follow what they recommend.

Incidentally, the keto diet has been shown to improve your chances of conceiving and improving your fertility (Mullens & Dr. Andreas Eenfeldt, 2019). So if you have problems conceiving, talk to your doctor about this and see if it works for you.

## *Post Pregnancy*

Once your baby is born, the real issue you're going to have to deal with is whether you should continue keto or not. As mentioned earlier, intermittent fasting is out of the question since producing milk and feeding your baby will call for additional calories and you should not be reducing your food intake (Mullens & Dr. Andreas Eenfeldt, 2019).

Also, for as long as you are nursing your child, you should not be in a caloric deficit. The reasons for this are the same as that with intermittent fasting. If anything, you should be eating at maintenance or more to meet your body's needs.

So how do you go about losing fat? Well, keto is an excellent option for this, since it will induce body recomposition, which is converting your fat into muscle. It will take longer since you're not in a deficit, but this doesn't mean you should not follow it. The only thing to keep in mind is that your carb intake should be higher than on a regular keto diet, around fifty grams or more.

The reason for this is, you will lose sugar via your breast milk, and you need to replenish it to keep your baby healthy.

## *Case Studies*

In 2015, the Swedish Medical Association published in their journal the case of a woman who suffered from severe ketoacidosis six weeks after giving birth (Mullens & Dr. Andreas Eenfeldt, 2019). She was able to recover, but doctors noted that her diet might have played a part in inducing the condition in the first place.

Ketoacidosis occurs due to prolonged periods of starvation or less than usual food intake and is exacerbated by stress and lifestyle changes. Given that the woman was following a low carb diet at the time, the stress induced by the pregnancy seems to have caused the condition in her.

She had been following the diet for a long time before giving birth, and after delivery, she suffered from symptoms of nausea, fever, and a complete lack of appetite (Mullens & Dr. Andreas Eenfeldt, 2019). Given the demands of breastfeeding her baby placed on her, it seems that she didn't eat enough food.

Now, the way this case was reported is a good illustration of how a lot of the media exaggerates and distorts basic nutritional messages. While the journal noted that the woman was following a low carb diet, the media exaggerated it as the cause of her condition, and thus created a myth (Mullens & Dr. Andreas Eenfeldt, 2019). While it's true that the low carb diet did contribute to the higher levels of ketones, thus making her more prone to ketoacidosis, it was hardly the reason for her condition.

Further examination, and indeed, the woman's statements confirm the fact that she was practically starving thanks to the lack of appetite. That being said, there is the theoretical chance of a keto diet not being compatible with breastfeeding (*Mullens & Dr. Andreas Eenfeldt, 2019*).

During the lactation process, as mentioned earlier, your body produces sugar for the milk and if you restrict your carbs too low levels, less than fifty grams per day, the stress could be too much for your body to cope with. Add to this the conditions of flu, like in the case with the Swedish woman. You can see how the low carb diet can bring about ketoacidosis.

The Swedish Medical Association reported five cases worldwide of ketoacidosis during the breastfeeding period, of which three were linked to starvation, and two were linked to low carbs (Mullens & Dr. Andreas Eenfeldt, 2019). Thus, as you can see, it's not entirely clear cut what the effect of the keto diet is on breastfeeding.

## *Recommended Course of Action*

Dr. Andreas Eenfeldt, the founder and CEO of Diet Doctor, suggests that women can follow the keto or low carb diet while breastfeeding, but to increase their carb intake to at least fifty grams per day (Mullens & Dr. Andreas Eenfeldt, 2019). While doing this, it is also a good idea to keep an eye out for symptoms of ketoacidosis.

These include nausea, fever, and abnormal thirst. Upon experiencing any of these, you should increase your carb intake significantly, and if the symptoms still occur, then you should consult a doctor immediately.

The key, as he points out, is not so much what you eat but how much you're eating. You should be careful to provide your body with enough calories, and as long as you're providing it with enough carbs, you don't need to worry as much about the macronutrients you're consuming.

Adding fruits to your daily meals is a great way to increase your carb intake, for example. Prepare for this as soon as you can, and you'll be just fine.

## *Tips*

It is best to get started on the diet before you get pregnant, ideally three or four months prior. Of course, not every pregnancy is planned, but this is the best scenario. Your doctor is also likely to recommend that you don't change your diet for fear of any complications so you can reap the benefits of the diet.

The next thing to keep in mind is that you should be eating at maintenance at the very least. It's a good idea to eat more than that and maintain a caloric surplus for safety's sake. Your body is going to go through the wringer soon, and you'll need all the energy you can get.

Making sure you drink enough water and eat your vitamins is a general advisory for those on keto but it applies doubly to you. Your body will shed a lot of water, and this causes a lack of micronutrients, especially electrolytes, which you need to replenish. While Gatorade and its ilk are okay occasionally, the added sugar in those drinks isn't good for the long term, as mentioned previously.

Don't keep your carb intake too low, and aim for at least fifty grams per day as mentioned previously. Also make sure you're getting enough fiber, either through food or via supplements. Keto does lead to constipation issues if you aren't getting enough fiber in your diet, so keep this in mind.

Make sure you're tracking everything, as will be explained soon in the tracking chapter. Try to maintain a journal and monitor your milk based on how many carbs you eat. You'll also be tracking your baby's measurements at this time, so as long as your child is growing at the expected rate, you're producing enough milk for them.

As always, follow your doctor's advice and keep them updated with everything that's going on. Most of all, relax and enjoy the feeling of new motherhood!

# CHAPTER 7:

# THE SUPPLEMENT GUIDE THAT
# WILL MAKE YOUR LIFE EASIER

Supplements are called as such for a reason. Your primary source of fuel should always be whole food, and you should never rely too much on supplements if you can manage it. Sometimes, this is tough. For example, if you're vegetarian, getting your quota of protein on the keto diet is going to be close to impossible.

Thus, you will need to supplement with a protein shake and BCAA. Generally speaking, I'm all in favor of protein supplements. There are, however, so many of them on the market that it makes your head spin.

In this chapter, I'm going to break down the supplements you need to have and the ones you can opt for, but they aren't all that necessary. I'll also list out the ones you don't need unless a doctor specifically recommends them. Given a large number of supplements that do exist out there, it is impossible to cover each and every one of them. If you see anything missing from here, you don't really need it in the first place.

So, let's begin by looking at the supplements you should have.

## THE MUST HAVES

The supplements in this category will help you across all three areas of the regimen, which is with intermittent fasting, the keto diet, as well as your workouts.

### *Protein Powder*

Protein powder comes in two forms: whey and casein. Whey protein is digested and released faster, while casein is a slower releasing protein. Given that you'll be fasting, it would seem the casein is the ideal choice. However, there isn't any significant difference between the two, and you're better off sticking with whey thanks to the greater options in terms of price, as well as flavor, it provides (Van de Walle, 2018).

Since milk is not allowed on the keto diet, mix your protein powder scoops with water and add some berries (which are allowed) to the shake. Generally speaking, it's best to consume protein both before and after your workout. Given the larger size of your post workout meals, focus on consuming the bulk of your protein shake portion before your workout.

If you're on the go and happen to be busy during the time you break your fast, a few scoops of protein powder will keep you full for some time. Don't make a habit of this, however, since this is not a meal replacement.

In case you're wondering, protein powder is not a steroid of any kind, nor will it cause you to bulk up magically. It is simply protein and is no different from what you'd get eating meat. Even if you're able to meet all of your protein targets through whole food, keep some lying around the house for an emergency. Sometimes, you'll be too tired to cook, and it's important to have a ready source of protein.

### Fiber

There are two kinds of fiber supplements available in the market: one in pill form and the other as powder. The opinion is divided as to whether the pills work or not. The powders, which are usually psyllium husk or flaxseed, certainly do.

I would say keep it simple and use the powder form.

Fiber is an essential part of the keto diet since the restriction on carbs results in fiber being restricted as well. A lot of dieters who begin the diet report either constipation or diarrhea, both these conditions are caused due to the higher than usual levels of protein most people are accustomed to eating.

Make it a habit of sprinkling your food with powder, they're usually tasteless and don't add anything significant in terms of calories. Be careful to stick to the recommended dosage though, or else you might find yourself pitching a tent in your toilet.

## *Magnesium*

How would you like me to give you a superfood that regulates your immune system, gives you energy and maintains your blood sugar levels? Well, it's plain old magnesium that does this, not some exotic superfood. An ideal dosage of magnesium is in the 200 to 400 mg range (Kubala, 2018).

Due to food being heavily processed these days, the vast majority of the population suffers from a deficit of magnesium, so this isn't just a ketogenic diet thing. Additional magnesium will help you combat irritability caused by low energy, aid in muscle recovery post workout, and enable you to sleep better.

Given what you'll be going through on this regimen, magnesium is something you should have stocked. In natural food, this is found mostly in avocados, spinach, and other greens.

## MCT Oil

MCT stands for medium chain triglycerides and is a form of fatty acid. MCT is mostly found in oils such as coconut oil. Coconut oil, incidentally, is one of the best sources for MCTs, so if you're cooking with this, you should be getting a steady supply of it.

MCTs are especially useful when breaking your fast because they are broken down quickly and give you an instant energy boost (Kubala, 2018). The flip side of this is the symptoms of nausea and diarrhea it can cause in some people.

Start with a small dose, half a teaspoon, and increase it gradually to see how your body adjusts.

## Omega 3

The omega 3 fatty acids DPA and EHA (both of which have incredibly long spellings which you can look up yourself) are essential for suppressing inflammation and lowering the risk of heart disease (Kubala, 2018). These should be consumed no matter what if you ask me.

The richest source of omega 3 acids is fatty fish, which are a big part of the keto diet. Fish oil supplements are widely available in the form of capsules. A word of caution though - a lot of these capsules are marketed as omega 3 but actually, contain vegetable oil inside them instead of fish oil.

Vegetable oil does have omega 3 in it, but in much smaller amounts than fish oil. Make sure you purchase the real thing. Generally, look for 500 mg of EPA and 1000 mg of DHA at the very least.

### *Multivitamin*

These supplements are a catch-all of sorts to make sure you fill in the gaps that are left from your regular diet. The most common deficiency is Vitamin D, so if you choose to supplement just that, that's fine as well.

## THE GOOD TO HAVES

The following supplements may or may not be of use to you depending on what you experience. Again, remember that none of these are substitutes for whole food and that you should be getting most of your nutrition from food instead of supplements.

## *Greens Powder*

Can you absolutely not stand eating green veggies? Don't like the thought of salads? Well, then a greens powder supplement is a good alternative. There are a large number of them available on the market. A pleasant side effect of this is that you will almost certainly get your fill of micronutrients by consuming this.

Can they be used as a like for like replacement for actual greens? Well, despite containing powdered spinach and wheatgrass, you should have some green veggies with all of your meals simply because it's better to eat whole food. However, there are no adverse effects of supplementing your greens like this in the long run.

## *Electrolyte Supplements*

During the initial stages of the keto diet, it is a good idea to keep a few packets of electrolyte powder handy in case you lose track of your fluid loss. After you adjust to the diet, you probably won't need them. The electrolytes you will need to replenish the most are sodium, potassium, and magnesium.

All of these can be found in spinach, avocado, and leafy greens. However, supplementing with this is also a good idea.

## *Branched Chain Amino Acids*

BCAAs are vital if you choose to perform early morning fasted training. While whey and casein protein do contain BCAA, they don't carry them in the amounts necessary to make a difference (Kubala, 2018). BCAAs are released quickly into your system and thus will help prevent muscle loss when you work out fasted. This is why it's better to use these instead of protein powder, which has other nutrients and calories when fasted.

BCAAs reduce muscle fatigue and aid in recovery post workout. While you cannot substitute these for protein powder completely, thanks to the calorie count, if you're getting your protein from whole food, then consuming BCAAs right as you end your feeding period is a good idea to minimize any muscle loss that might happen.

## *Creatine Monohydrate*

Creatine is perhaps the most researched exercise supplement in recent years. As far as aiding your workout performance, nothing beats creatine. Do you need it for a ketogenic diet or IF? Well, not really. However, if you're serious about improving your workout performance, then it's a no brainer.

As far as costs go, monohydrate is one of the cheapest versions of creatine available, and you can purchase it in various forms, as a powder, pills, or liquid. Each of these is just as effective, so you won't be losing out by choosing one over the other (Kubala, 2018).

## Caffeine

Along with BCAA, this belongs in the must-haves for people who wish to carry out fasted training. Either in the form of pills or as a morning cup, coffee will get you going if you feel lethargic. A common supplement that mimics caffeine is marketed under the category "fat burner." These give you a boost of energy similar to caffeine, but without the side effects or addictive properties.

Understand that caffeine by itself doesn't burn any fat. It merely gives you a shot of energy that gets you working harder, and this is what burns calories and fat. If you're working out after meals, then there's probably no need for this. However, some people feel the need for a boost pre-workout. Incidentally, a pre-workout protein shake will give you a good boost as well, so don't think you need to rely on caffeine solely.

## Probiotic Supplements

The keto diet, incidentally, is excellent for those who suffer from a leaky gut and poor digestion (Kubala, 2018). During the transition period, though, you are likely to suffer from some discomfort. Probiotic supplements will help ease this.

Also, if you follow any low carb diet for a long time, your gut bacteria will die out, and you might see an increase in food allergies and such.

You can choose to either consume these in powder form or through food. The best whole food sources are anything fermented like sauerkraut or kimchi. Be careful of the added sugar in kimchi, though, and watch your carb intake with these options. The best sources of probiotic bacteria are yogurt and kefir, but these are ruled out thanks to the sugar in them. Greek yogurt is a fantastic keto option, however, and as long as you watch your carb intake, this will work well.

If you want to go the supplement way, then there are several gut health powders out there. I try to stick to whole food as much as possible, and I feel supplementing probiotics may be unnecessary.

Just remember that over the long term, you will need to add probiotics to your diet to ensure proper gut health.

## OVERRATED STUFF

Given the popularity of keto and IF, several supplements are being marketed that, frankly, have no earthly use. They come wrapped in fancy packages with fancy names and are marketed by so-called 'authorities.'

Before you get seduced by one of these, remember that fasting has been around since ancient times. Keto has been prescribed since the early 1900s to patients. There was no need for a ton of supplements back then, and there's no need for a ton of them now.

Below is a list of stuff you don't need to worry about, not all of them are useless, mind you. Some of them are overkill for someone who's starting and are a waste of money. Supplementing these will give you fewer returns for your effort than merely cleaning up your diet and making sure you follow the guidelines listed previously.

Exogenous ketones - There's no proven research that these work.

HMB (beta- hydroxy beta- methyl butyrate) - This works, but those who lift weight at expert levels will find more use for this than beginners or intermediates.

Beta-alanine - Same as above, it prevents fatigue but nothing that a good night's rest won't cure.

Proteolytic enzymes - Seriously, just eat good food.

Molecular Hydrogen

Adaptogenic herbs - Do you like adding rosemary, basil, etc. to your food? Yes? Then you're covered.

Fat burning 'stimulants'- This is separate from fat burners mentioned above. These are marketed as somehow mobilizing your fat for better burning, whatever that means.

Binders for biotoxins - An IF supplement, these bind biotoxins together to help reduce adverse reactions during the fasted state. If that sentence made sense to you, do let me know!

Mass Monster XXXXL etc. - You've seen these products at your local GNC. While they're mostly marketed at guys, there are a few women who end up buying these thanks to their fat burning promises. Again, eat good food, and you'll be fine.

This is not a comprehensive list, of course. As I said, there are so many of these things floating around; it's impossible to cover all of them. Stick to the lists in this chapter, and you'll be fine.

# CHAPTER 8:

# TRACKING RESULTS AND WATCHING THAT FAT FALL **OFF!**

Tracking is the final essential element of your fat loss plan. Think of it this way: whatever you don't track, you cannot improve. You'll have to track a lot of things, from your food intake, your weight, your exercise performance and so on.

Well, I'm here to tell you that it's a lot simpler than it seems. Sure, at first you're going to feel as if you're facing a mountain of stuff, but over time, a lot of this is going to become second nature. Much like how you'll be able to approximate the calories in a meal by looking at the serving portion, you'll be able to track a lot of stuff, such as your weight, by just checking in with how you feel.

Tracking also helps you get over the dreaded fat loss plateau which every single dieter hits. There's a specific way for you to blast past this, and I'll show you how in this chapter.

So, let's dive right in and look at the things you need to track from a workout perspective!

## WORKOUT PERFORMANCE

We start with the most straightforward stuff to track: your workout performance this is oddly, something you won't see a lot of gym goers do. Usually, people got to the gym and lift random stuff and go back home, wondering why they aren't making progress.

Always carry a notepad and pen with you to the gym and write down your numbers. Here's what you need to be recording.

### *Exercise Plan*

What is your workout plan for the day? Which exercises will you be performing for how many sets and reps? What is the weight you'll be lifting? As you perform each exercise, record whether you could carry it out or not. A plan will come in handy when you begin stalling at certain weight levels and need to figure out how to move past them.

### *Exercise Form*

Your form can be classified as a 'nice to have' to be honest. You can ask someone to take videos or pictures of you as you progress. This way you'll be able to monitor yourself for any mistakes in form or technique you might inadvertently be making. You don't need to record every single workout session. Once a week should be more than enough.

# PHYSICAL MEASUREMENTS

## *Weight*

This one's obvious really. You need to measure your weight since this is the best way to make sure you're achieving progress. Now, a lot of people know how to measure their weight but go about interpreting the results in the wrong manner. Here's what you need to do.

Weigh yourself every day at the same time. So, if you weigh yourself first thing in the morning before brushing your teeth, do it at that exact moment. Don't weigh yourself the next day after having a glass of water, etc. Note down this number.

After a week, calculate the average of your measurements and note down this number. This number will be your average weight for that week. The next week, calculate the average weight. Now, compare the weekly average numbers. If the numbers are decreasing healthily, you're good. If not, you need to make some changes.

Far too many people worry about their daily weight numbers. Your weight, daily, will fluctuate for a variety of reasons either due to water retention, release, stress, and so on. If you get caught up with them, you'll be missing the forest for the trees. So take a step back and only concern yourself with the weekly numbers.

### Waist Size

Here's another big one. Your weight decreasing is a good indicator of weight loss, but remember, fat loss is what we're trying to achieve. So measure your waist every day and average those numbers out. As long as you're losing inches, you're fine.

I recommend taking a loose measurement of your waist since this is a more accurate picture. Think of yourself as a tailor measuring yourself out for a new dress. Don't feed your ego and suck your belly into an extreme.

### Other Measurements

If you choose to, you can measure your biceps, hips, etc. as well, but there's no benefit to these beyond a feel-good factor. If you have the time, go ahead and do so.

## Pictures

Take pictures of yourself! This is going to be your before/after record, and it's vital for you to see the progress you're making visually. Stand in front of the mirror at the same spot at the same time every week and take a snap of yourself. The best time to take a picture is after you wake up.

You'll be in a fasted state, and your body is not likely to be bloated from food, so you'll get a better morale boost from these pictures.

## Body Fat Percentage

Whether you need to measure your body fat percentage or not is up for debate. There's no denying that measuring it is the best way to track your progress. However, the amount of effort and money it takes to get an accurate measurement makes estimating your body fat percent a better return for your time spent.

There are several ways to measure your body fat percentage. I've listed them in order of least time consuming to most.

The U.S Navy Estimate - This estimate is good enough for the armed forces, and hopefully, it's good enough for you. You need to measure your neck and your waist along with putting your body weight and height into an online calculator. You'll then receive your body fat percent. Is this accurate? Well, it's an estimate for a reason. However, it is accurate to within a percentage point or two from personal experience.

Calipers- Measuring yourself with calipers is relatively straightforward. You pinch a fold of fat on your waist, and seven other body areas into the caliper and the resultant measurement corresponds to a particular body fat percentage. How accurate is this? Well, not very, to be frank. You can expect close to the same level of accuracy as the previous method, especially if you have a lot of fat to lose. It gets more accurate the leaner you get.

BIA Scales- Bioelectrical impedance scales send small shots of current through your body and measure the resistance encountered. Such machines are widely available, and you can carry this out in your home. Note, though, the measurements are most accurate on an empty stomach. Fluid intake significantly distorts the results.

DXA Scan- This process consists of taking two X-Ray scans of your body while you lie down. It is non-intrusive and doesn't take very long. A plus point of this is you receive information about your bone density along with details of fat concentration in your body.

Hydrostatic Weighing- File this under impractical but accurate. This method involves submerging yourself in water after exhaling as much air as possible and weighing yourself when submerged. No, don't do this in your bathtub. Hydrostatic Weighing requires specialized equipment and is usually available in research centers and don't do this at home alone.

Bod Pod- Equally impractical to everyone except professional athletes, the bod pod gives you the most accurate fat percentage based on a technique called air displacement plethysmography. Well, it's a big word, so it must be accurate!

If you can afford them, BIA scales are the best investment. As long as you're above 30% body fat, you don't need to worry too much about tracking this. Once you get below 30%, it makes more sense to track this since progress will be much tougher and you'll need to measure everything as much as possible.

### *Body Mass Index*

Here's a twist in the tale for you. Don't bother measuring the BMI. The BMI is a simple calculation of your weight divided by your height. The resulting number is a good indicator of health. The problem with the BMI is that it isn't very accurate or reflective of health when you become lean and have more muscle mass. For instance, a lot of athletes rank as obese on the BMI standard, which is a bit ridiculous.

If you're carrying a lot of fat it is reflective, but do you need to track this? Not really, since you're tracking other numbers which give you a far better picture. The BMI is one of those mainstream numbers that get bandied about often but makes no sense.

## DIET MEASUREMENTS

In addition to the food prep items I mentioned in the relevant chapter, you're going to need something vital for your success: a food measuring scale. Trust me, do not skip buying one. It is essential you have this ready and know how to use it. A simple one will do - there's no need to get all fancy with it.

### *Food Portions*

How many grams of meat are you going to cook? What about your veggies? How much oil are you pouring out?

It's going to seem like overkill at first, but the time you spend initially learning to measure quantities out is going to reap your huge rewards. By doing this at home, you'll find it easier to size up your portions in restaurants and know how much you should eat ideally.

### Calorie Tracking

This one is essential, as well. There are several apps out there, with myfitnesspal being the most popular. I use a free account at fitday.com to track everything I eat. Input what you're eating throughout the day, before you eat it, and then check to see if it matches your desired calorie count.

You can also use several apps for this and program your target calorie count for the day into the app. The best thing to do is to enter everything you plan on eating for the day when your day starts. Doing this is not as difficult as it sounds since a lot of your meals will be either precooked or be derived from the same base. It'll just be a matter of adjusting one or two entries every day.

### Activity Tracking

You could track the amount of energy and calories you're burning throughout the day, but frankly, measuring your body weight is just a better method, despite being slower. People got by just fine without these trackers, and I've never seen a huge need for them unless you happen to be a fitness nerd (not that there's anything wrong with that).

# KETO TRACKING

### *Ketosis Tracking*

Tracking your blood or urine ketone level is essential to check whether you're in ketosis or not. This is especially the case if you've indulged in some extra carbs for your cheat meal. You should purchase urine strips, which are easily available to check for this.

These are invaluable when you first adopt the keto diet and are transitioning into it. Check for ketosis regularly and make sure you stay there. Use it to determine your ideal number of carbs. Some people cannot handle less than fifty grams simply due to biological restraints.

Ketone testing strips will solve a lot of issues for you, so go ahead and buy them.

## A SAMPLE TRACKING ROUTINE

Now that you know the various things you need to track, how do you put it all together? Well, here's a sample tracking routine for a typical day once you've adjusted to the keto diet and are regularly working out.

As you wake up in the morning, before doing anything else, you weigh yourself and note down the number. Then, you measure your waist using a measuring tape and note that down as well. If this is the seventh day of the week, then calculate the average of both numbers and compare them to the previous week.

If the number has risen, then you must have eaten more than you think the past week. Make a mental note to adjust your portion sizes down a little bit. Even better, recalculate your portion sizes based on a total caloric intake that is 250 calories less than your current intake level.

If the number is decreasing healthily, you're all good. If it's decreasing by more than 1.5 pounds per week, then you're eating far too few, and you're losing muscle as well. So, increase your intake by 250 calories in your calculations and figure out your new portion sizes.

Once this is done, you can choose to take a photo of yourself if this is the designated day. Pack your food for the day according to your schedule. If you're cooking food, then measure and cook the relevant quantities. Make sure you're carrying some nuts with you instead of snacks as you step out.

Keep track of the water you're consuming throughout the day, aiming for at least four liters of water. Before visiting the gym, make sure you have your fill of protein and consume less than sixty percent of your total calories for the day before this. Also, if you haven't already, write down which exercises you need to perform, the weight and sets and reps.

At the gym, execute your workout plan and record your numbers. If you stall, follow the stall procedure according to the strength training programs, Starting Strength or Stronglifts, as mentioned previously. Once you leave the gym, have a meal within an hour of leaving.

As the time of your feeding period draws to a close, check whether you've hit all your goals for the day. Prepare for bed and carry out the same plan the following day.

This is all there is to it: not some magic or special tasks you need to carry out. Hopefully, now you can understand why I've said that losing fat is a simple and repeatable process that anyone can follow on the IF plus keto protocol.

All this tracking has a secondary purpose, in that it will help you blast past the dreaded fat loss plateau. Let's take a look at how to overcome this.

## THE FAT LOSS PLATEAU

If you've followed any diet regimen at all, you'll be aware of the fact that the fat loss plateau exists and getting past it is a significant challenge. With regular diets, this plateau occurs relatively early in the process, once the initial water weight has been shed. After a few weeks of progress, you begin to find that your weight stays the same despite continuing to do the same things.

Well, thanks to implementing intermittent fasting, you will not only lose the water weight but also not experience a plateau at all. To understand this better, we need to know why the plateau occurs in the first place. Well, if you recall from previous chapters, we saw how to lose weight, you need to be in a caloric deficit.

Now, here's an added wrinkle. Remaining in a caloric deficit is great right up until it stops working. This is because of your basal metabolic rate, or BMR, which we looked at previously, also changes as you lose fat. Your BMR reduces by almost the same amount as the percentage of body fat you lose with studies as far back as 1917 showing that a 30% reduction in calories is accompanied by a 30% reduction in BMR (Fung, 2018).

Thus, as your BMR decreases, your caloric deficit vanishes and therefore you stop losing fat. So what do you do now? Eat even less? Well, not quite. This is harmful because the lower your BMR drops, the lower your internal body heat drops as well, and beyond a certain point, it doesn't make sense to keep cutting calories until all you're eating is a few shards of lettuce.

The key to continued fat loss is insulin. Insulin is what your body uses to extract energy from carbs. If your carb intake happens to be high, your body keeps the insulin level high and thus the body is primed to burn food that comes from outside, as opposed to looking within and burning the fat inside (Fung, 2018).

Hence, to continue losing fat, we need to keep our insulin levels low and steady. Keto and intermittent fasting are the best ways of doing this. By eating a diet that's low in carbs and fasting for an extended period, we're telling our bodies that food is not forthcoming as easily as before.

Therefore, it has no option but to look inward and start burning the fat that is within us. This is why on IF+keto, which effectively combines both insulin lowering methods, you won't encounter a fat loss plateau. The question arises, though - is it even necessary to maintain a caloric deficit to lose weight? After all, it looks like insulin is the key to everything, so why bother eating less?

Well, understand that losing fat is a two-part process comprising of what you eat and how often. Thus, the more food you eat, the greater the levels of insulin you will be producing within you. To kickstart your body into burning the fat that is stored within you, you need to eat less. Once your body gets used to the fact that nothing is going to be fed to it for sixteen hours, it adjusts and starts burning internal fat for its purposes (Fung, 2018).

Therefore, think of the caloric deficit as the initial impetus that moves your fat loss snowball down the hill. As it rolls further and further, it gets more prominent, and it sustains itself through momentum. However, a snowball can't get started without that initial force. That's what the caloric deficit is.

Focus on keeping your insulin levels low, and you'll continue to lose weight healthily. You won't need to worry about your caloric deficit after the initial few pounds you lose. IF and keto are excellent methods to keep you on track, but here are some other pointers to lower your insulin:

Avoid foods that cause energy spikes like energy drinks or too much chocolate. Dark chocolate is fine, but don't go wild with it.

Exercise regularly and engage in resistance training, which is just strength training. Hopefully, now you can see why I devoted so much time to the strength training section in this book.

Reduce stress by meditating, relaxing, and monitor your stress levels. This is because when you're stressed, your body seeks to release more energy, and this produces more insulin to mobilize whatever energy source is present (Fung, 2018).

## MENTAL STRENGTH

So it's 6 PM on a Friday, you're done with work, and your friends are pestering you to join them early. However, you still have a workout left, and you know that you'll have to limit your nighttime calorie intake thanks to your fast. If this sounds like a nightmare scenario to you, well, unfortunately, you're going to be facing it a lot more than you think.

Your willpower is like a muscle. The more you use it, the more it strengthens. However, like any muscle, it gets weak from overuse and a lack of rest. The key to staying the course and being mentally strong is to conserve your mental energy. This is why it is so essential for you to cut stress as much as possible and even reward yourself through cheat meals once a week.

These function as stress relievers, but again, don't run away with yourself and overdo it. Have a single piece of that brownie, instead of the entire batch. By exercising your will power during these cheat periods, you're actually building up your reserves. If you feel the need to binge or overeat, I suggest you stop dieting and take a step back.

Taking a step back seems contrary to all other advice out there, which tells you to keep pushing no matter what. Well, the reality is that you can only push for so long. Lasting change comes when you implement change in small, bite-size portions and integrate them into your life. How do you do this? Well, firstly, it's about building good habits, and secondly, it's about implementing these new habits in small steps.

If you are someone who doesn't stir off of her couch all day and watches TV all the time and considers walking to the strenuous bathroom exercise, well, no matter how hard you try, you will fail. It's not that such a person is incapable of change. It's just that the change is too big for their system to bear.

Our brains love inertia or remaining in the state they currently are in, and this is because it means processing information is easy, and there's not much stress involved. The key to implementing change is to introduce it in small, almost imperceptible steps so that your mind doesn't revolt and before it realizes it, you've installed a new habit.

Going back to our example of the terminally lazy person, the first step would be to ask herself, is walking for ten minutes a day really that bad? Probably not. So, get up and walk! Next, is reducing the TV watching time by a single show and reading a book instead that difficult? No? Well, do it then.

By repeatedly performing these actions and continually pushing as far as comfortably possible, our boundaries grow and before you know it, you'll have no trouble implementing change. If you struggle to maintain discipline, this is a symptom that the change you're trying to achieve is too much. I'm not talking about momentary feelings of laziness that hit everyone.

No, I'm talking about a constant, almost violet reaction towards something you'd like to do. If you find going to the gym excruciating, forcing yourself to go there is only going to use up your willpower, and you'll have none left to follow your diet. The key to staying strong, you see, is to use your willpower as sparingly as possible.

Another good way to motivate yourself is to inject some emotion into the proceedings.

- Why do you want to lose weight?

- Why are you doing this?

- What will it bring you?

Imagine having what you want and focus on how it feels. Focus on how good it feels and how your life changes. Even if it's a ridiculous sounding thing, it doesn't matter. This is your world! You get to imagine whatever you want.

Every day, remind yourself of why you're doing this and how it will feel when you achieve what you want. By doing this, you'll slowly and surely get there.

# CONCLUSION

Intermittent fasting allied with the ketogenic diet remains the best and fastest way to lose fat and get that sexy body you've always dreamed of having. While it will seem daunting at first, remember that once you get into it and start working things out, you'll find it gets a whole lot easier.

For starters, we looked at intermittent fasting and why it's so beneficial. By narrowing your feeding window to eight hours, you're forcing your body to reduce its insulin stores whereby it begins to burn your internal body fat. A great way to kick start this process is by maintaining a caloric deficit. Although you can try to do this without a deficit, it'll take you longer and frankly, 500 calories are not as much as you think.

To boost the efficacy of this process, we add the ketogenic diet into the scheme of things. Under the rules of the keto diet, you will be restricting the amount of carbs you consume to under thirty grams or even fifty grams if that suits you better. There will be some problems when transitioning, but using the methods in this book, you'll navigate the keto fog easily. It won't always be pleasant, but hey, it won't last too long either.

Remember to always consult your doctor before starting any diet regimen. This doubly applies if you have any medical conditions or are pregnant. Even nursing mothers ought to talk to their doctors first. The best way you can reap the benefits and get rid of the eventual post-baby weight gain is to adopt the keto diet before your pregnancy. While fasting during pregnancy and the nursing period is not a good idea, the keto diet can help you immensely.

There are many pitfalls of adopting this way of eating, so make sure you review all the do's and don'ts in the appropriate chapter. Remember to relieve your stress as much as possible. This whole regimen works because it is predicated on you not harming yourself. Admittedly, it can sometimes be tough to differentiate between you being lazy and something just being entirely unsuited for you, but keep working on it and you'll be able to tell the differences easily.

Your mental state is something you should guard, and the best way to use your willpower is to use it conservatively. Which means if any situation is getting out of hand, stop, and take a few steps back. Doing this will help you reassess things and chart a better, improved course. This applies to your diet as much as the work you put in at the gym.

Do your research to determine which strength training program works best for you. It will be intimidating at first, but as I said, those gym bros respect you for venturing into their zone, given the complete lack of females in that area. So go ahead and represent!

Make sure you learn proper techniques and form before increasing the weight to prevent injury, which will be worse with compound movements. Follow a strength training routine and build your strength levels up to an intermediate standard according to the program you choose to follow. Once this is done, you can switch to a higher rep program.

Go easy on the cardio since strength training itself will take a heavy toll on you. If you choose to do HIIT, then skip the steady state cardio and do it as a separate session, instead of at the end of your workout.

Supplements will make your life a whole lot easier, but remember that whole food should be your primary fuel source. The only exception to this is protein for vegetarians and vegans, where you can substitute protein powder for all your protein needs. Again, some calorie counting is initially required to determine how much you ought to eat, but once you begin losing fat, you can maintain this level of eating.

Make sure you include lots of fiber via food and supplements in your diet, to prevent constipation, which often occurs. Magnesium is another supplement that will help you immensely. The easiest way to get all of this is to have lots of leafy green vegetables. These are pretty low in calories, so you can have lots of them as well.

Tracking is what will make or break your results. You need to track your calories initially but can maintain your portion sizes as time goes on. Meanwhile, make sure you track your weight, waist size, and any other measurements you choose. Remember to track your progress in the gym as well to deal with stalls. Also, remember to monitor your ketone levels via test strips to figure out if you're in ketosis or not.

If you experience any symptoms of dizziness or excessive fatigue, increase the amount of food you're eating. If your symptoms persist, seek your doctor's advice.

Remember to prepare before adopting this new method of diet and exercise. It is not easy enough for you to jump in and expect to swim. It takes work, but with the right preparation and determination, you'll achieve everything you want. Remind yourself of this every time things get tough, and you feel like quitting.

Feel free to take an occasional break to clear your head. If things are getting to be too much for you, skip a few gym days instead of skipping your diet rules. However, remember to come back to your rules and keep track of your progress. Use this to motivate you and improve your life.

Finally, remember that I went through this struggle as well. I was once in your position, at a complete loss as to what to do and how to go about doing it. I certainly don't believe I'm a person blessed with anything extraordinary. All I did was take this step by step, as I've laid it out here. I guarantee that if you follow this plan, you will see results within thirty days flat!

I hope you've gained a new understanding of fat loss and dieting by reading this book. Please do let me know what you think by leaving a review!

I wish you all the best of luck and love in the world for your journey! It's going to be great girl. You got this!

# REFERENCES

Antunes, F., Erustes, A., Costa, A., Nascimento, A., Bincoletto, C., & Ureshino, R. et al. (2018). Autophagy and intermittent fasting: the connection for cancer therapy?. Clinics, 73(Suppl 1). doi: 10.6061/clinics/2018/e814s

Berkhan, M. (2015). The Leangains Guide | Leangains. Retrieved from https://leangains.com/the-leangains-guide/

Bjarnadottir, A. (2018). The Beginner's Guide to the 5:2 Diet. Retrieved from https://www.healthline.com/nutrition/the-5-2-diet-guide

Daly, M., Paisey, R., Paisey, R., Millward, B., Eccles, C., & Williams, K. et al. (2006). Short-term effects of severe dietary carbohydrate-restriction advice in Type 2 diabetes-a randomized controlled trial. Diabetic Medicine, 23(1), 15-20. doi: 10.1111/j.1464-5491.2005.01760.x

Eat Stop Eat Review (2019): A Legit Diet For Weight Loss? Or Fake Fad?. (2019). Retrieved from http://www.healthvi.org/diet-reviews/eat-stop-eat-review/

Foster, G., Wyatt, H., Hill, J., McGuckin, B., Brill, C., & Mohammed, B. et al. (2003). A Randomized Trial of a Low-Carbohydrate Diet for Obesity. New England Journal Of Medicine, 348(21), 2082-2090. doi: 10.1056/nejmoa022207

Fung, J. (2018). Understanding Obesity. Retrieved from https://medium.com/@drjasonfung/understanding-obesity-f233fbb38dc1

Gunnars, K. (2017). Intermittent Fasting 101 — The Ultimate Beginner's Guide. Retrieved from https://www.healthline.com/nutrition/intermittent-fasting-guide#effects

Kubala, J. (2018). The 9 Best Keto Supplements. Retrieved from https://www.healthline.com/nutrition/best-keto-supplements#section7

Mullens, A., & Dr. Andreas Eenfeldt, M. (2019). Is Low Carb and Keto Safe During Pregnancy? - Diet Doctor. Retrieved from https://www.dietdoctor.com/low-carb/pregnancy

Van de Walle, G. (2018). What's the Difference Between Casein and Whey Protein?. Retrieved from https://www.healthline.com/nutrition/casein-vs-whey

Zauner, C., Schneeweiss, B., Kranz, A., Madl, C., Ratheiser, K., & Kramer, L. et al. (2000). Resting energy expenditure in short-term starvation is increased as a result of an increase in serum norepinephrine. The American Journal Of Clinical Nutrition, 71(6), 1511-1515. doi: 10.1093/ajcn/71.6.1511

Zhou, W., Mukherjee, P., Kiebish, M., Markis, W., Mantis, J., & Seyfried, T. (2007). Nutrition & Metabolism, 4(1), 5. doi: 10.1186/1743-7075-4-5

www.ingramcontent.com/pod-product-compliance
Lightning Source LLC
Chambersburg PA
CBHW031136020426
42333CB00013B/406

* 9 7 8 1 9 5 0 9 2 1 1 4 0 *